# NATUROPATHIC JOINT MOBILIZATION

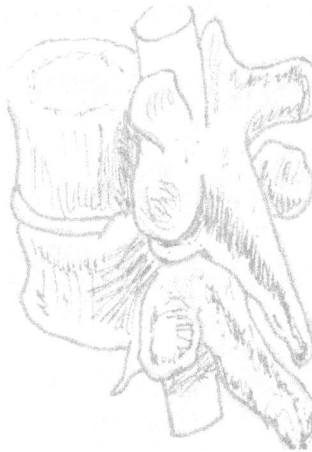

C. P. Negri, OMD, ND

**Infinity Health Care**

NATUROPATHIC JOINT MOBILIZATION
By C. P. Negri, OMD, ND

Photography by Jeanne-Marie Fabian
With illustrations by the author

Printed in the United States of America.

ISBN: 978-1-7372929-4-4

Care has been taken to confirm the accuracy of the information presented in this work.  While the subject matter of this book contains generally accepted practices in several licensed healthcare professions, many are not accepted in the practice of mainstream medicine and do not represent the consensus of medical opinion at this time.  The reader should be aware of this and the author and publisher are not responsible for errors or omissions, or for the consequences from the application of the information in this book and make no warranty, express or implied, with respect to its contents.  It is the responsibility of each provider to ascertain the current status of, and possible complications from, any and all procedures that are given or recommended.

also by C. P. NEGRI:

Green Medicine
Naturopathic Treatment of Blood Pressure
Naturopathic Treatment of Emotional Illness
The Negri Manual of Natural Medicine, Vol. I and Vol.II
Why Natural Therapies Work (and How to Make Them Work Better)

# DEDICATION

To
## Dr. William von Peters

For keeping the legacy of
**Dr. Frederick Collins**
alive

◇

# CONTENTS

## FORWARD

It has to be noted that so much that was of worth and taught in natural medicine has been lost in the past 100+ years. Among the lost teachings and techniques are the Naturopathic and old Osteopathic spinal and joint adjustment methods. Both have gone into obscurity, with a great deal of the techniques and movements completely lost to the body of knowledge of man. The "old timey" docs and med school professors who knew or taught the techniques to previous generations and my generation of natural docs, are all dead!

In the present day, Chiropractic is looked to for spinal adjustment and some DCs also do joint manipulation. But the spinal adjustment techniques and various methods (such as Gonstead, "Hole In One" or Subluxation Specific, Pierce-Stillwagon, Directional Non Force Technique, Activator, Cox, and the many, many other variations of Chiropractic adjustment), differ entirely from the mechanics and execution of both the Naturopathic and the old Osteopathic techniques.

With the collective profession forgetting its prior teaching subjects, such as the Osteopathic cranial and sacral adjustment techniques taught in Dr. William Sutherland's *The Cranial Bowl* textbook, (which is markedly different and produced markedly better results than today's Cranial Sacral Technique), the profession and professionals have lost valuable tools from their armamentarium.

Fortunately for the current practitioners of natural medicine, there remains one physician who was thoroughly schooled in the Naturopathic adjustment technique. His mastery and application of the various spinal and joint manipulation treatments, combined with a half century of practice, has made him likely the world's leading if not only exponent of the old methods. He now passes that expertise and its clinical pearls to a new audience, a new generation of natural and alternative physicians. It is my hope that this work will serve to preserve and promote once again the widespread use of these tried and true methods for relieving human suffering.

Enjoy the learning and the doing!


William Wong, N.D., PhD

*Dr. Wong is a former instructor of physical medicine at Southwest College of Naturopathic Medicine (now known as Sonoran University).*

# PREFACE

In addition to all the other natural modalities that came to comprise Naturopathy, manual therapy was a front runner. Most naturopaths used some kind of manual therapy as well as their other chosen tools. In reviewing the earliest literature on naturopathic approaches to joint mobilization, it is painfully obvious that the old texts were of little real value in *teaching* any of the maneuvers, separate from the actual classroom instruction. Sometimes the instructions are incomprehensible, due to mistyping "left" for "right", or failing to mention that the operator is standing behind, not in front of, the patient. It is not that the old instructors had a lower standard; even the most up to date 21st Century textbooks have been found to be riddled with errors.

What we present here are the major methods of joint mobilization, arranged in order of simplicity and reliability; upright and also reclining. The instructions are fully illustrated and the intent is to *teach,* not simply catalogue technics.

Before we examine these in detail, a bit of history: Spinal manipulation did not originate with Osteopathy or Chiropractic; it was not only previously established in the Far East but also in the the Bavarian region of Europe where the first notable exponents of Nature Cure resided. However, Naturopathy in its early days of organizing in the US was populated by doctors who were also osteopaths. Because of this factor (and because it is in the nature of the naturopathic field to adopt whatever drugless method is of value), joint mobilization became a major tool of the classical ND. The earliest technics adopted by them were osteopathic in origin. As the field progressed, some uniquely naturopathic technics were developed.

In time, the osteopathic profession was split from within, between those wanting to remain a drugless, manipulative profession and those who wanted parity with medical doctors. Traditional, drugless Osteopathy largely disappeared within a short time. But this coincided with the rise of its offshoot, Chiropractic.

Many chiropractors began to be dual trained in Chiropractic and Naturopathy, and DC / NDs were common. Chiropractic methods, which differed slightly from osteopathic methods, crept into naturopathic practice. Over time, the chiropractic profession became hostile to the naturopathic profession and the bond was broken.

But naturopathic schools today most often employ a chiropractic doctor to teach manual medicine[1]. The end result of this is that a lot of the historical technics are being forgotten. Ironically, they are among the safest and require the least training to be effective.

This book is an attempt to correct that loss, while not attempting to be a comprehensive text. You will find a suggested reading list at the end.

C.P. Negri, OMD, ND
2024

---

[1] Likely because chiropractors are plentiful, and most osteopaths today don't use manual medicine.

## MOBILIZATION CATEGORIES

For a good grounding in naturopathic joint mobilization, it is necessary to have three categories of technics at your command:

1. Soft tissue technics
2. Mobilization without impulse
3. Mobilization with impulse
    a. Long lever technics
    b. Short lever technics

Massage and manipulation have been used since ancient times as remedial agents. Massage needs no description for the average reader, although the various methodologies of massage therapy can be as different as night and day. The application of the hands can range from a soft, sensual stroke to a penetrating pressure to a rhythmic percussion.

### Soft tissue technics

From the naturopathic viewpoint, the body's normal metabolism is subverted by various elements that interfere with proper functioning. Waste products from altered metabolism or from inflammation can create blockages to eliminative pathways, involving blood vessels, nerves, and the viscera themselves. A primary mechanical interference is the appearance of adhesions. Not only localized waste, but also localized inflammation, trauma, or scar tissue from surgery can cause adhesions to form.

Naturopathy has long had a group of manual technics known collectively as "Bloodless Surgery". Its primary use is in breaking adhesions to allow proper circulation. While this is most often employed with the abdominal contents, which is beyond the scope of this book, it is pertinent in discussing the joints. The shoulders and hips particularly are prone to adhesions, and the technic for dealing with them should be discussed.

Palpation of adhesions requires some practice, but it is well worth the effort to be able to spot these limiting factors and deal with them, when they can nullify your best attempts otherwise. When examining a joint, pay attention to the condition of the overlying soft tissues and not just the range of motion. The tissues may feel normal and smooth until you reach a specific site. Then you will feel a band or rope-like texture in the fascia. Sometimes it presents as a series of knots. After trauma and strains, the fascia in the region sometimes maintains a buckled shape, and without a mechanical correction, remains as an adhesion.

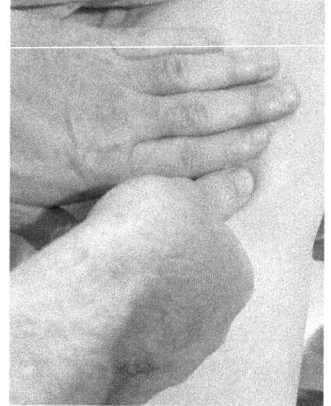

The Bloodless Surgery technic most successful for dealing with adhered tissue employs both hands. The five fingers of your non-dominant hand are placed flat at the site, and you give a deep pressure (equally distributed across all fingers) on the order of 10-15 pounds. You can test this on a bathroom scale until you get the "feel". The purpose of this pressure is to immobilize the offending tissue.

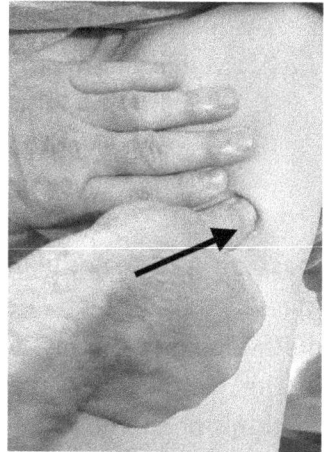

The other hand is employed as the "scalpel". The fleshy part of the thumb is placed in contact with the index finger of the immobilizing hand, and pressed downward. Next, slide the thumb back and forth, using the edge of the index finger as the guide. Maintain the downward pressure throughout. You may feel a tearing or sudden relaxation of the connective tissue as a fibrous band snaps, and there may be an audible snapping sound. Generally, such elastic tissue being torn does not cause pain. The thing to remember is that this technic is contraindicated if there is severe pain experienced from simply palpating the site. If that is the case, lightly palpate and feel if there is a pulsation under the surface. If so, the local congestion must be reduced by other means so as not to cause internal hemorrhage by this maneuver.

The effect of this treatment continues to build over a week's time. It may take several sessions to achieve the results desired.

## Mobilization without impulse

Joints can have their range of motion increased by various deep pressures on the connective tissues, or guided range of motion maneuvers, or induced isometric contractions, or traction on the limbs. In such cases, it is called **mobilization without impulse**.

 

1. **PROM** (Passive Range of Motion)

Passive Range of Motion differs from active range of motion in that it is not an action taken by the patient (Active Range of Motion) but rather a guiding of the body by the operator while the patient relaxes. It is helpful to first ask the patient to move the limb (or torso) as far as possible in the direction specified. When the physiological barrier is reached, i.e., no more movement is possible, the operator takes over control and asks the patient to relax. Then the motion is continued smoothly and slowly and held for a brief time at the maximum range.

2. **PNF** (Proprioceptive neuromuscular facilitation)[1]

Proprioceptive neuromuscular facilitation is a common method for increasing range of motion in a joint. It is commonly referred to as "PNF". It is also known as "Muscle Energy Technic" in massage and osteopathic circles. But it has been known since the 1940s, when it was developed by Dr. Herman Kabat and used for treating the residuals of polio and multiple sclerosis. Naturally, a non-drug therapy for neuromuscular diseases was not implemented widely. It later came to be called the "3 S Method". This stood for "Scientific Stretching for Sports", thus removing its use for serious maladies. But, like all great advances, it never died and has come to be adopted in physical therapy.

PNF has been studied for its application in sports performance, and several theoretical mechanisms have been put forth as to why it works. It is likely a combination of mechanisms that enable PNF to achieve increased range of motion, but the mechanisms do not concern us here. It is a very simple technic (a *principle*, actually) and is easily learned.

There are a few ways to perform PNF, but all depend on stretching a muscle to its physiological limit. This initiates the Golgi tendon reflex or "inverse myotactic reflex". It is a protective reflex that relaxes the muscle to prevent injury. The Golgi tendon organs

---

[1] Often referred to as "Muscle Energy Technique".

within the tendon of a muscle (insertion or origin) send a signal to the brain that the muscle is about to tear. The brain in return sends a message to the muscle to relax.

Often, PNF can restore normal ROM without using any mobilization with impulse maneuvers, and therefore should be tried first. In any event, it will relax a muscle enough that an impulse move will be much easier.

Here is the basic technic:

1. **Locate the major muscle involved in a restriction of motion.** We will use the example of a restricted side bending of the cervical spine on the left side. The suspicious muscles would be the Trapezius, Sternocleidomastoid, and Scalene muscles on the right side.
2. **Relax and lengthen those muscles by stretching the patient's neck** in left side bending. Stabilize the right shoulder while using the other hand to slowly side bend the head.
3. **When the barrier is reached, ask the patient to try to move the head back against the resistance of your hand.** This isometric contraction should last about seven seconds.
4. Tell the patient to relax the tension, breathe in, and breathe out. When the patient breathes out, **use the anchoring hand to again guide the head toward the side.** You will likely find that the second stretch will go farther than the first. If the normal range of motion is not achieved, repeat the process two more times.

With a little thought as to the kinesthetic workings of the joint, one can use this method to isolate any problem muscle.


## Mobilization with impulse

Mobilization can also be a very precise application of force to a specific site that is designed to move a bony structure. A thrusting motion is made to accomplish this. When this is the case, it is called **mobilization with impulse**.

Contemporary authors are now in the habit of referring to non-impulse methods as "mobilization" and impulse methods as "manipulation". This deviation from the traditional terminology does not, in the author's opinion, convey any greater understanding of the matter. But it does suggest to the reader's mind that "manipulation" belongs to one level of practitioner. Everyone recognizes that once you "own" a word or title, you can stifle competition from outside. Because of this rather obvious self-serving language, we will retain the term **mobilization** in this work. After all, mobilizing the joint is the main point, and one needs only to consult a dictionary to see the broad definition of "manipulation".

Manipulation, in therapeutic terms, has been vaguely described as the therapeutic application of manual pressure or force. This is fine, since manipulation can be applied to soft tissue and thereby becomes a form of, or outgrowth of, massage. This would be mobilization without impulse.

Joint mobilization *with* impulse is another matter. It is defined as a "passive manual maneuver during which a three-joint complex is taken past the normal physiological range of movement without exceeding the anatomical boundary limit".

The defining characteristic of spinal mobilization for most people, especially those familiar with Chiropractic, is the dynamic thrust—a sudden force that causes an audible release (*cavitation*, the process that produces the "pop" sound) and is intended to increase a joint's range of motion[2].

This "popping" kind of maneuver, however, is only one of five grades of joint mobilization. Each grade produces different effects by selective activation of mechanoreceptors in the joint, as the following will describe.

---

[2] Studies have concluded that cavitation or popping is not essential for a maneuver to be therapeutically successful.

# Grades of Joint Mobilization

## Grade I:

- Activates Type I mechanoreceptors that have a low threshold and respond to very small degrees of tension placed on the tissues

- Activates cutaneous mechanoreceptors

- If stimulation is oscillatory, it will selectively activate rapidly adapting mechanoreceptors such as Meissner's and Pacinian corpuscles.

Examples:
- Swedish massage,
- Bowen Therapy,
- (light) Shiatsu,
- Mechanical vibration

## Grade II:

Examples:
- Lymphatic drainage,
- Naturopathic "Bloodless Surgery" method

- Similar to Grade I.

## Grade III:

Examples:
- Deep tissue massage,
- Naprapathic soft tissue technic,
- Nimmo Technic,
- Neuromuscular Therapy,
- Shiatsu,
- Reflexology

- Similar to Grade II, but selectively activates an increasing number of muscle and joint mechanoreceptors as the tissues go into resistance, and less of the cutaneous mechanoreceptors as the slack of the subcutaneous tissues is taken up.

## Grade IV:

- Similar to Grade III, but containing a more sustained movement at the end of range of motion, which is often near the resting or neutral position. This activates the static, slow-adapting Type I mechanoreceptors, whose resting discharge increases in proportion to the degree of change in joint capsule tension.

Examples:
- Myofascial Release,
- Passive range of motion,
- High amplitude / low velocity movement seen in Asian bodywork
- PNF (proprioceptive neuromuscular facilitation), also known as "Muscle Energy Technique"

## Grade V:

- The classic high velocity, low amplitude (HVLA) thrust that is practically synonymous with spinal "manipulation". The joint is positioned near to its end range of motion during this type of joint manipulation, and an impulse is applied to carry it just beyond the functional limit but within the anatomical limit. Now referred to in some circles as HVT (high velocity thrust).

Examples:
- Osteopathic Manipulative Therapy,
- Chiropractic Manipulative Therapy,
- Naturopathic Manipulative Therapy,
- Oriental Medicine Manipulative Therapy,
- Japanese *Sekkotsu* Therapy

Soft tissue manipulation is performed by a number of different types of massage therapists in the wide range of bodywork methods available.

Many people do not associate the practice of joint mobilization with naturopaths and Oriental medicine practitioners, but these two groups have also historically used these techniques. However, in the U.S., there are two specialties that have been most associated in the public's mind with joint manipulation: Osteopathy and Chiropractic. Most people have never heard of Naprapathy, but it also rightly belongs in the pantheon of manipulative professions (although it does not depend on HVT), and some naturopathic doctors have studied Naprapathy also.

### Differences in approach

Osteopathic technics and naturopathic technics both favor "long lever" maneuvers; the patient's limb (or torso, or head) is often used as a lever to produce passive motion in a selected region. When impulse is applied, multiple joints may be moved during such a procedure. It does not isolate one spinal segment and it stretches the paraspinal muscles more than "short lever" maneuvers.

Chiropractic technics favor "short lever" maneuvers; the hand is used to make thrusts to a contact point on a specific process, typically at a 90 degree angle. The "short lever" is the spinous process or transverse process or lamina that, when forced, creates a change in the articulation of the joint with its neighbors. Assessment is made of where to make the thrust, and which direction, angle, and degree of force will best correct the position of the joint.

Naturopathic mobilizations tend to be less harsh overall than the manipulations most seen today. The osteopathic-origin maneuvers that naturopaths inherited separate the facet joints during the process; many chiropractic maneuvers compress ("lock") them. Naturopaths, like early osteopaths, perform mobilization with the targeted area more or less under traction, rather than compression. Chiropractors, under the theory that their job is to correct subluxations, view manipulation more like corrective surgery. Thus, they call their manipulation an "adjustment". Thrusting to the spinous processes is common.

At the risk of being repetitious, the author feels that naturopaths in the present time should refer to their maneuvers as **mobilizations** (with or without impulse), not as "adjustments" (a chiropractic term), or "manipulations" (an osteopathic term). Also, as a point of clarity, naturopaths refer to the **restriction** as being the problem to be corrected, as opposed to the "vertebral subluxation complex" in chiropractic terms, or "somatic dysfunction" in osteopathic terms[3]. The naturopath should strive to correct the restriction in not only the joint's mobility, but the restriction of the local tissues in eliminating toxic waste, as mobilizations have a decided impact on connective tissue.

## What is "impulse"?

The founder of my Alma Mater, First National University, used to describe it as "that unique spontaneity of movement". It is a sudden continuation of a joint's movement once it meets the physiological barrier; that is, the point of restriction. While the joint has an anatomical range of motion (i.e., the physical range that a joint can naturally move), a restriction of that full range limits the movement to what is called the *physiological* range of motion. A barrier is met in attempting to move the joint toward the normal end point of motion. The patient may experience discomfort when reaching the physiological barrier, but often not. At that point, a measured impulse is made to drive the joint past the barrier (but not as far as the anatomical end range). The impulse may take the form of a sudden rotation, a thrusting motion, a change in the central axis of the spine or limb, or sometimes more than one. It is performed with, as Dr. Frederick Collins termed it, "that unique spontaneity of movement". That is, suddenly and precisely. It is designed to briefly gap the joint by about 1/8 inch.

---

[3] Formerly referred to as "lesion".

8

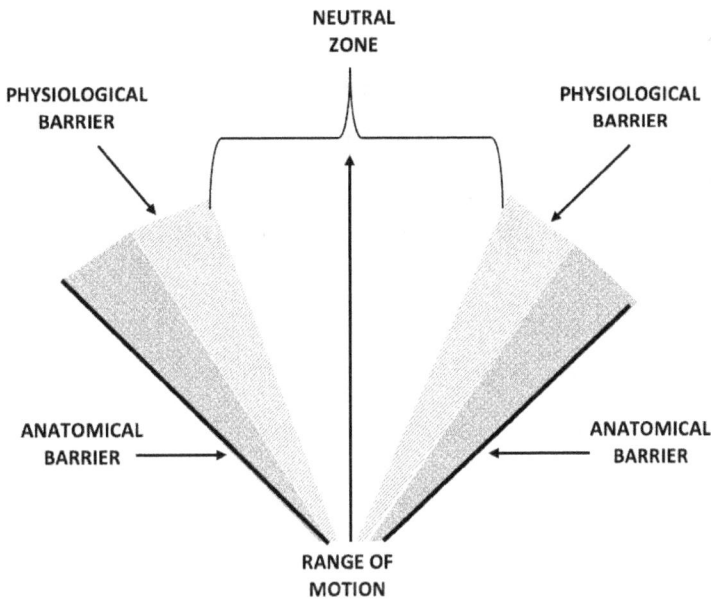

NEUTRAL
ZONE

PHYSIOLOGICAL
BARRIER

PHYSIOLOGICAL
BARRIER

ANATOMICAL
BARRIER

ANATOMICAL
BARRIER

RANGE OF
MOTION

It is essential that the naturopath develop assessment and palpatory skills so as to be able to recognize when the physiological barrier is met (rather than waiting for the patient to say "It won't go any farther").

It is also essential to coach the patient with explanations and commands such as "Breath out", "Relax", etc., in order to minimize muscle tension during the procedure. Never attempt to apply impulse to someone who is tensing up or fighting your efforts. For this reason, preparatory methods such as hot packs, muscle stimulation, diathermy, mechanical vibration, etc. are often used before mobilization. And, if possible, soft tissue technics such as PNF (covered in a later section) ideally should be employed before a mobilization with impulse, in the hope that they can resolve the problem first and impulse technics are not needed. While certainly not unknown in osteopathic and chiropractic practice, this is a distinctive feature of *naturopathic* manual correction.

# CONTRAINDICATIONS FOR SPINAL MOBILIZATION WITH IMPULSE

## Screen your patients!

- Patients currently taking fluoroquinolone drugs (Ciprofloxacin, etc.)
- Patients currently taking blood thinning drugs
- Acute whiplash
- Disc herniation with neurological deficit (numbness, paresis)
- Down syndrome
- Carotid artery disease
- Cauda equina syndrome
- Cervical myelopathy
- Osteoporosis
- Localized inflammation
- Ankylosing spondylitis
- Avascular necrosis
- Spina bifida, and other malformations of the spine
- Infection (osteomyelitis, meningitis, tuberculosis of the bone, etc.)
- Osteomalacia
- Bone tumor
- Aortic aneurism
- Intracranial hypertension
- Bleeding disorders (hemophilia, blood thinners)
- Spinal cord compression
- Fractures, of course

# SECTION TWO

## ASSESSMENT

Three methods of assessment are used in Naturopathic Joint Mobilization:

1. Inspection
2. Palpation
3. Kinetic tests

There is a fourth, sometimes necessary, method and that is testing for impaired nerve conduction. This is beyond the scope of this book.

There are three aspects of a patient's body that must be assessed:
- Asymmetry (Is one shoulder higher? Are the iliac crests level?)
- Range of motion (ROM) of the joint under observation
- Tissue texture (skin, fascia, muscle, ligament)

Asymmetry and range of motion are assessed by visual inspection.
Tissue texture is assessed by palpation and percussion.

### Asymmetry

This is a visual evaluation, and the anatomical landmarks for assessing this are illustrated in this book for each region of the spine and extremities.

### Range of motion—kinetic testing

Likewise, the normal anatomical range of motion (ROM) for each joint is illustrated in each section of this book. In motion testing, a part of the body is either moved actively by the patient or passively by the doctor.

### Tissue texture

Palpate lightly to evaluate the skin, dragging it a short distance vertically and horizontally. Notice if the tissues seem tighter or looser in a certain direction.

After getting a feel for skin elasticity in the region, gently apply more pressure and evaluate the underlying fascia. With a little practice, you will be able to identify any thickening that has been established; fascial bundles can often be found between adjacent muscles.

Now increase the pressure deeper to focus on the muscle. See if you can feel the individual fibers. Move your fingertips both longitudinally and transversely, differentiating between smoothness and roughness. The most common finding in an area of restriction is hypertonic tissue. The patient usually describes it as "It feels tight."

As you practice, the palpatory skill gained reveals what osteopaths call "motion sense"—you get an accurate idea of how restricted a joint is, and whether there is hypertonicity or hypermobility present.

**Spinal Examination**

Inspection, percussion, and palpation are the major methods for examining the spine. Adjunct methods include thermographic measurement, electrical skin resistance measurement, and dolorimetric readings (applying standardized pressure to see where there is tenderness). Imaging ranges from X-rays and MRIs to contour analysis and thermograms.

Of all these, palpation is the most important. The position of the patient must be changed accordingly as the examiner checks for different types of abnormalities. For example, lateral curvatures are best detected when the patient is bending forward, often while sitting. Rigidity of the spinal column, thickening of the spinal ligaments, degree of separation of the spinous processes—all are better detected with the patient in a lateral recumbent position. Other postural abnormalities are spotted more easily when the patient is standing normally.

# Detecting bony causes of restriction

There are six directions in palpating and recording restrictions caused by malposition or subluxation, known by the mnemonic PARLSI.

| Term | Abbreviation | Anatomical | Meaning |
|------|------|------|------|
| Posterior | **P** | Dorsad | Toward the rear |
| Anterior | **A** | Ventrad | Toward the front |
| Right | **R** | Dextera | Toward the right hand |
| Left | **L** | Sinistra | Toward the left hand |
| Superior | **S** | Cephalad | Toward the head |
| Inferior | **I** | Caudad | Toward the feet |

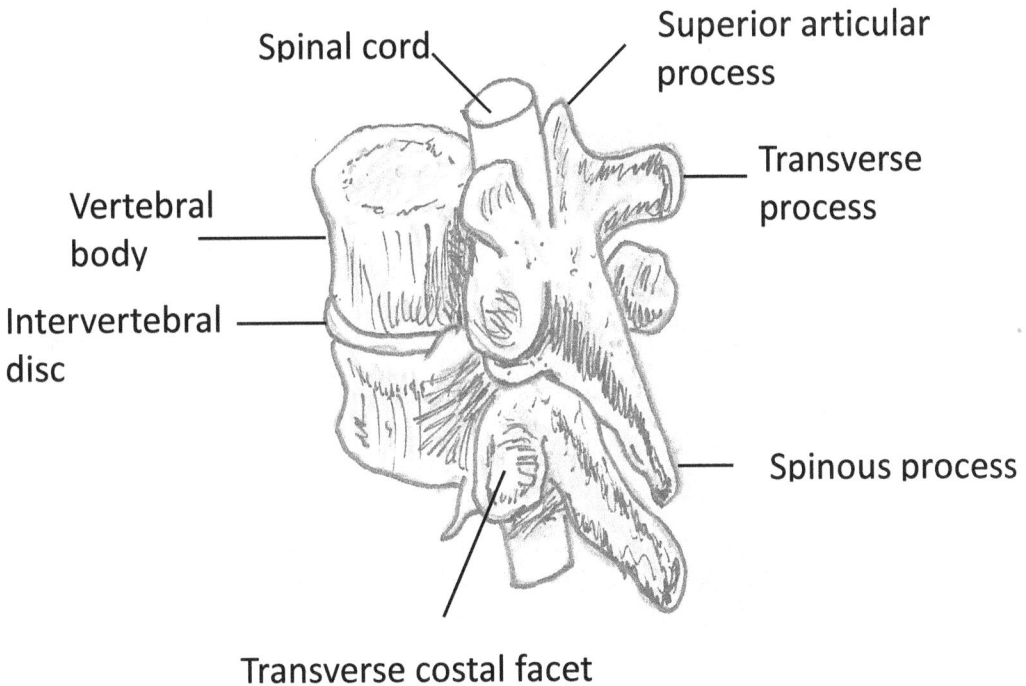

Spinal cord

Superior articular process

Transverse process

Vertebral body

Intervertebral disc

Spinous process

Transverse costal facet

## Palpating a posterior malposition

A posterior malposition is posterior *relative* to the vertebra above and the vertebra below it. As your fingers slide down the spine, the posterior vertebra is the one which

Juts out in the path of the fingers, forcing them to describe follow outward curve, like a bump in an otherwise smooth road.

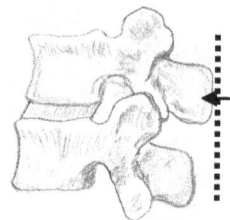

## Palpating an anterior malposition

The anterior vertebra is perceived by the fingers as a depression, causing the fingers to dip into the indentation. Anterior malposition or subluxation is not typically recorded in the examination notes because of the difficulty in reducing them, with the exception of the cervical spine and the fifth lumbar vertebra.

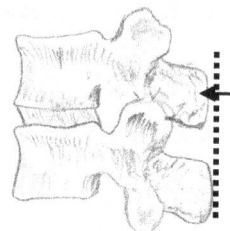

## Palpating a superior malposition

A vertebra is considered superior when its spinous process is nearer the vertebra above than the one below. It requires a measuring of relative distances.

## Palpating an inferior malposition

By the same token, a vertebra is considered inferior when it is closer to its neighbor below than to its neighbor above.

It will occur to the reader that other information needs to be gained in order to accurately diagnose the type of malposition. For example, is it a superior T5 or an inferior T6 causing the gap? The presentation of the spinous processes can suggest either. The problematic vertebra will be the more tender one, and thus simplify your analysis.

## Palpating left and right malposition

The right or the left malposition is assessed by running the tips of the fingers down the sides of the spinous processes, index finger on one side, middle finger on the other. It alerts you to rotation of the whole vertebra, more often than any other malposition.

## Side bending restrictions

In the diagram at right, the patient is made to side bend to the left. While the vertebrae at top and at bottom remain plumb, the middle segment shows a left side bending restriction. The arrows indicate the spinous processes. Note that the transverse processes are tilted on the restricted vertebra.

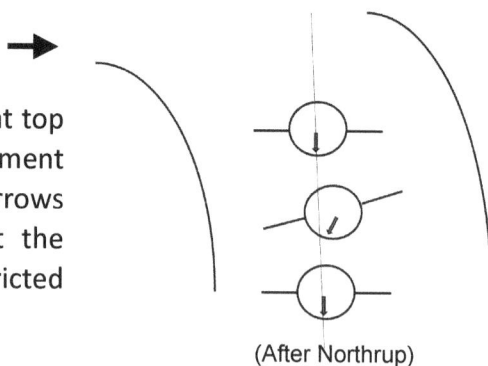

(After Northrup)

14

> Restriction (naturopathic)
> Somatic dysfunction (osteopathic) }
> Subluxation (chiropractic)
>
> Defined by the World Health Organization as:
> "A lesion or dysfunction in a joint or motion segment in which alignment, movement integrity and/or physiological function are altered, although contact between joint surfaces remains intact. It is essentially a functional entity, which may influence biomechanical and neural integrity."

## Palpation Technic

Palpatory procedure begins with the axis, because the atlas is evaluated in a different manner, covered in the chapter on cervical mobilizations. The hands are used in a different manner when palpating the spine in a sitting position than if the subject is prone. But regardless, the index, middle and ring fingers are used in a gliding motion down the spine. With the middle finger registering the tip of the spinous process (SP), let the other two fingers contribute information by touching the sides of the SP. It is advisable to shift from side to side, changing hands intermittently, as you palpate each vertebra in turn. The reason for this is that impressions of the two hands may be different and bring more clarity into your assessment. Secondly, it reduces fatigue. It is valuable for the naturopath to develop an ambidextrous palpation ability.

## Counting SPs
Establish a silent count as you begin at the second Cervical (axis). This is the first spinous process below the occiput. Smoothly glide the fingers downward over the tips and along the sides of the spinous process. Count silently to yourself "C2" and continue down the spine through the thoracic region and the lumbars until you reach the sacrum, without interrupting your motion. If you raise your fingers from their contact during the count, you simply begin again at the second Cervical. It is ,unfortunately, not likely you will replace your hand accurately once it is removed. Resume the count and make note of any anomalies found at a particular spinal segment and mentally note the vertebra. It should be entered into your progress notes for that day. The sacrum is easily identifiable when it is reached.
Have the subject stand and crouch behind, placing the middle finger of each hand on the crest of the ilium. Then move the thumbs toward the midline. Thumbs should be level with the middle fingers, with the horizontal line corresponding to the space between the third and fourth lumbar vertebrae. Variations in this line should be noted.

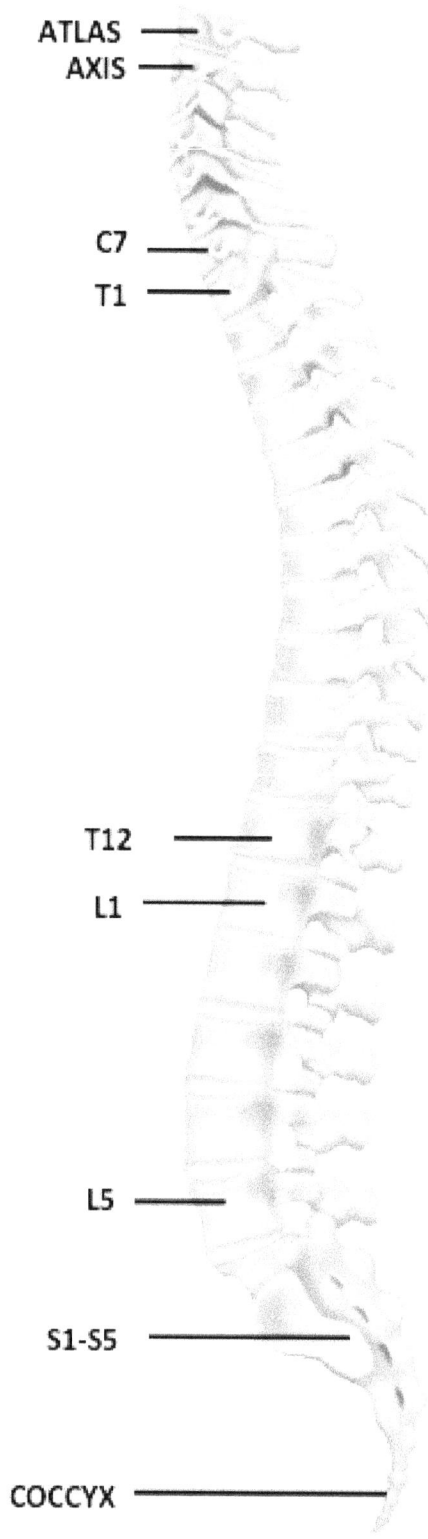

ATLAS ——

AXIS ——

C7 ——

T1 ——

T12 ——

L1 ——

L5 ——

S1-S5 ——

COCCYX ——

## Troubleshooting

There are several common problems encountered in counting vertebrae:
- Inaccessibility of the third Cervical, which lies closely beneath the spinous process of the second and cannot be readily felt at the SP. Sometimes it is more palpable if malpositioned, and sometimes simply due to a larger than usual bony structure.
- Sometimes an anterior fourth or fifth Cervical which may be missed unless the head is flexed far forward or the transverse processes examined directly.
- Adipose tissue covering the spine is a common impediment.
- Occasionally, you may find an extra vertebra such as an L6.
- Excessive cervical or lumbar lordosis can make evaluation difficult. In such cases, palpate the cervicals with the subject's head in flexion, and the lumbars with the body leaning forward with the subject's elbows resting on the knees.

But the development of the touch sense is most important in mastering spinal examination, and only practice brings it about.

## Charting

Record your findings in this manner (See next page):

**Column One** shows the spinal segments where a restriction has been detected.
**Column Two** shows the direction of malposition.
- The first designation, if pertinent, is P or A (excepting the atlas, which can only be L or R, S or I). Note that palpation is not the only way of determining this. When restriction is found in flexion movement of the spine, the spinous process is posterior or P. If motion is restricted in extension, it is Anterior or A.[1]
- A lateral deviation to the left or right, or a rotation to the left or right, is then written as L or R. (Some practitioners prefer to designate rotation as R and the side as a lower case "l" or "r", which would render a C4 right rotation as C4 Rr.)
- The proximity of the vertebra to its neighbor is recorded next, designated as S or I for superior or inferior. This may be evidence of narrowing disc space.

With this schema, a vertebra found to be posterior and more deviated to the right and slightly inferior, would be written as PRI. The right rotation is evident in that the spinous process is observed to be left of the midline.
**Column Three** records the corrective maneuver used. This is a movement that propels the vertebra in an opposite direction from its deviation[2].

---

[1] Some educators will render P as "F" (for flexion) and A as "E" (for extension), since the vertebra is not always literally posterior or anterior. The presence of flexion or extension restriction is obvious from kinetic testing of ROM.

[2] As Ashmore states in *Osteopathic Mechanics* (Journal Pub. 1915), "The articulating surfaces must retrace the the path they took in their displacement."

Below are examples, not a prescription.

| Site | Restrictions | Corrective Maneuver |
|------|--------------|---------------------|
| C2 | LI | Collins hook |
| C4 | PLS | Cervical rotary |
| C7 | LI | Prone rotation |
| T9 | RS | Seated lift |
| L4 | L | Lumbar roll |

Some doctors place emphasis on one finding as being more important to the case than another, and thus underline the the finding on the record.  It is a matter of personal preference.

The obvious advantage to charting in this manner is that you have a record of your findings for ongoing therapy sessions that preclude a full palpatory exam every time. One can accurately apply manual therapy without relying on memory and without wasting time.  Do, however, confirm that your findings of that day correspond to the record, and any changes should be noted for future sessions.

Patient name

DOB                    Date

**NOTES**

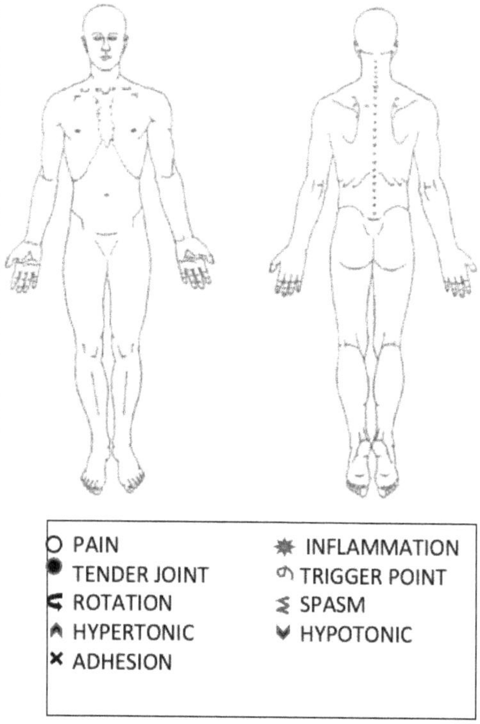

| | |
|---|---|
| O PAIN | ✴ INFLAMMATION |
| ● TENDER JOINT | ↷ TRIGGER POINT |
| ↰ ROTATION | ⩽ SPASM |
| ⋀ HYPERTONIC | ⋁ HYPOTONIC |
| ✗ ADHESION | |

It is important to state at this point that, over the years, many schools of thought have arisen as to the "best" way to perform spinal mobilization.  In chiropractic circles the tendency has been to become more and more specific; the exact malposition and its location, orientation, and the *exact* angle and depth of force in order to correct, must be decided before acting.  Some go as far as predicting the exact number of millimeters the vertebra has to move, and new technics have evolved to accomplish this.  The chiropractic profession has strained to present its totally scientific and up-to-date approach to throw off the old claims of "pseudoscience" by the medical establishment.  Sometimes this has resulted in an unnecessary complicating of the material.

This is somewhat analogous to academia producing more and more in-depth material to be studied, to keep raising the standard (and the college's profit) for a degree.

**Naturopathic mobilizations recognize the *fact* that when a therapeutic action is taken, even in a non-specific way, the patient improves because the innate drive to heal is natural.**

Leo Spears, DC, though he was a chiropractor, manipulated like a naturopath.  He stated it beautifully:

> Instead of being a fault it is a *virtue* to move a number of vertebrae with each thrust, but excessive force should not be applied in order to do so.

Likewise, in Chapter 9 of *The Buxton Technological Course,* A.G.A. Buxton, DC, wrote:

**Adjusting Every Vertebra**

One of the strange notions conceived by many chiropractors is the adjusting of a major subluxation, with total disregard for the minor.  It is as evident as an axiom in mathematics that one vertebra bears a relation of juxtaposition in every sense of condition to an adjacent vertebra, varying only in degree to the major malalignment, and the doctor who cares to give a thorough spinal correction will look after the minor as well as the major, however slight the abnormality.

Therefore, the reader should not be overwhelmed with the specificity spelled out in some of this material.  While trying to be as accurate as possible, the veteran doctor routinely mobilizes in a general manner and just as routinely gets great results.

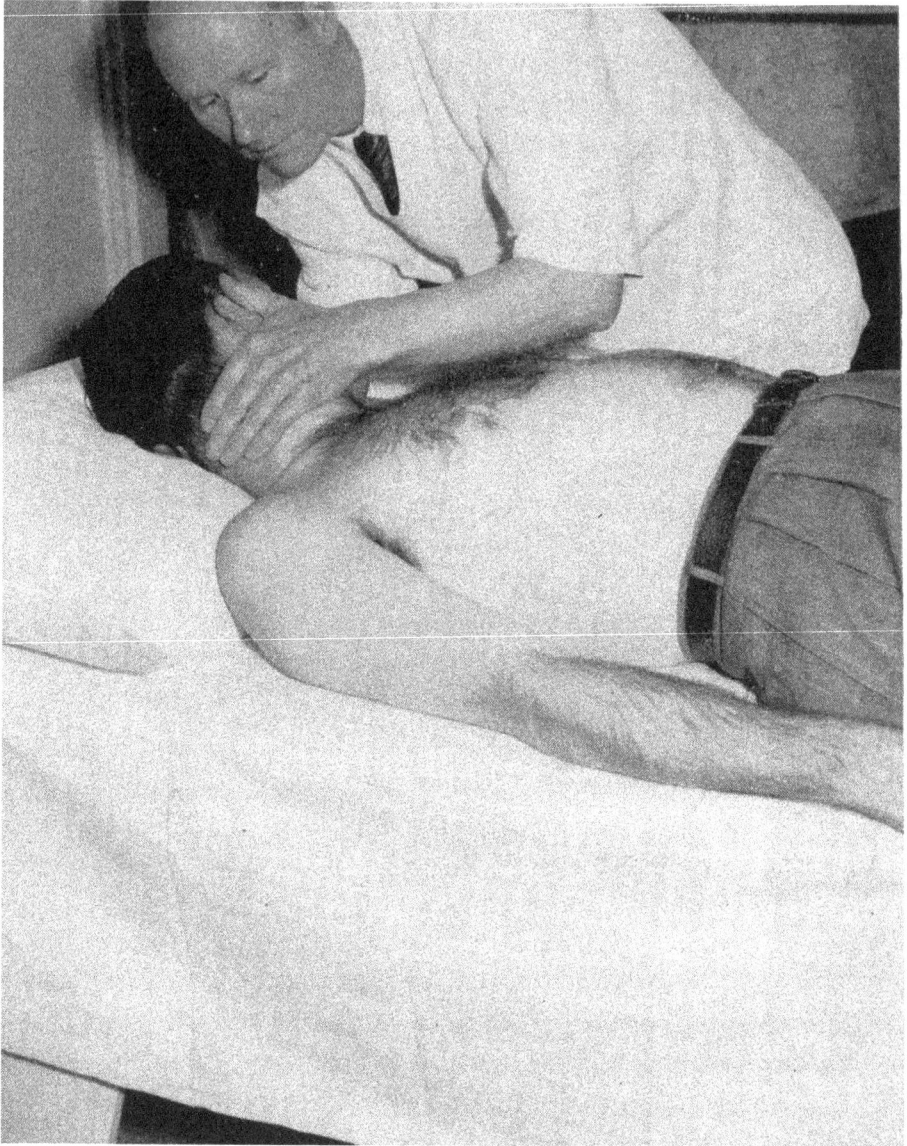

Leo Spears, DC, mobilizing the cervicals in a posture not common to chiropractors, but common to naturopaths

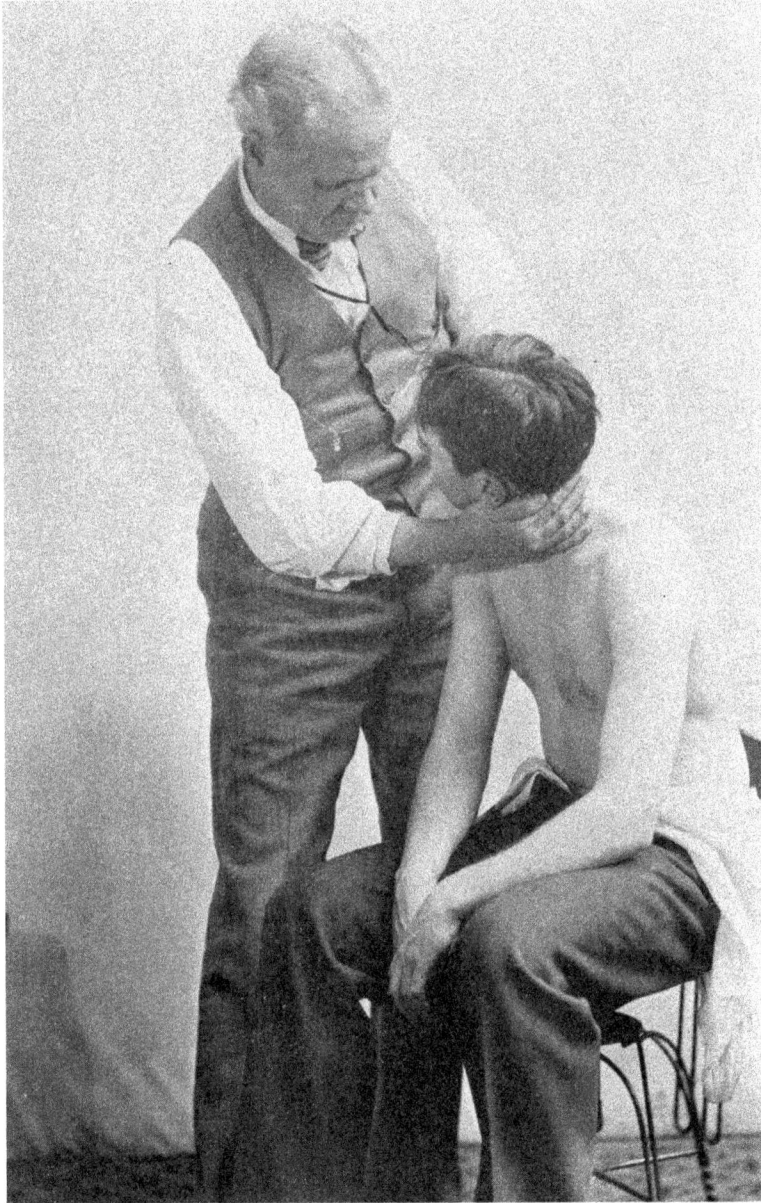

Buxton

# SECTION THREE

## CERVICAL MANEUVERS

The cervical spine is the natural starting point for discussing mobilization of the spine. The author hesitated to introduce it first of all regions in this book because of the typical uneasiness of naturopaths new to the practice of mobilization with impulse. It is perfectly acceptable to skip to the next section and begin working on the thoracic spine until one is more comfortable with the idea of mobilizing the neck. But the issue of vertebral artery dissection must be discussed.

The highly-publicized instances of upper spinal manipulation causing a tearing of the vertebral artery have made many uneasy. This unease is due to the dramatic reports of safety issues, although "authorities" have reported such vastly different adverse event numbers from one in 50,000 manipulations to one in 5.8 *million*[1]! While this is a legitimate concern, there seems to be little agreement on just how often such injuries occur, considering the *millions* of cervical adjustments made by chiropractors every year[2].

Nevertheless, soft tissue technics and non-impulse mobilizations are recommended as first-line maneuvers for cervical spine problems, with impulse technics reserved for cases that do not resolve completely with the non-impulse methods.

**The simplest way of avoiding adverse events is to pre-screen the patient. Rotate and extend the neck, and if vertigo or any sensory disturbance occurs, do not use mobilization with impulse.**

As was stated earlier, naturopathic mobilizations are inherently safer in the cervical region because the spine is under traction rather than compression, and the spinous processes are not impacted. Moreover, the cervical vertebrae are not mobilized in extension, as is sometimes done in Chiropractic.

---

1 Haldeman, et al., 2001: Risk factors and precipitating neck movements causing vertebrobasilar artery dissection after cervical trauma and spinal manipulation. *Spine*, 24(8), 785-794
Margery, et. al., 2004: Pre-manipulative testing of the cervical spine review, revisions and new clinical guidelines. *Manual Therapy*, 9(2), 95-108

2 I know of no comparison between this and, say, the adverse events during and following spinal surgery. I am sure, though, that no one is going to call for suspension of spinal surgery, even if the numbers surpass cervical manipulation.

C1 (Atlas)

C2 (Axis)

C3

C4

C5

C6

C7 ("*Vertebra prominens*")

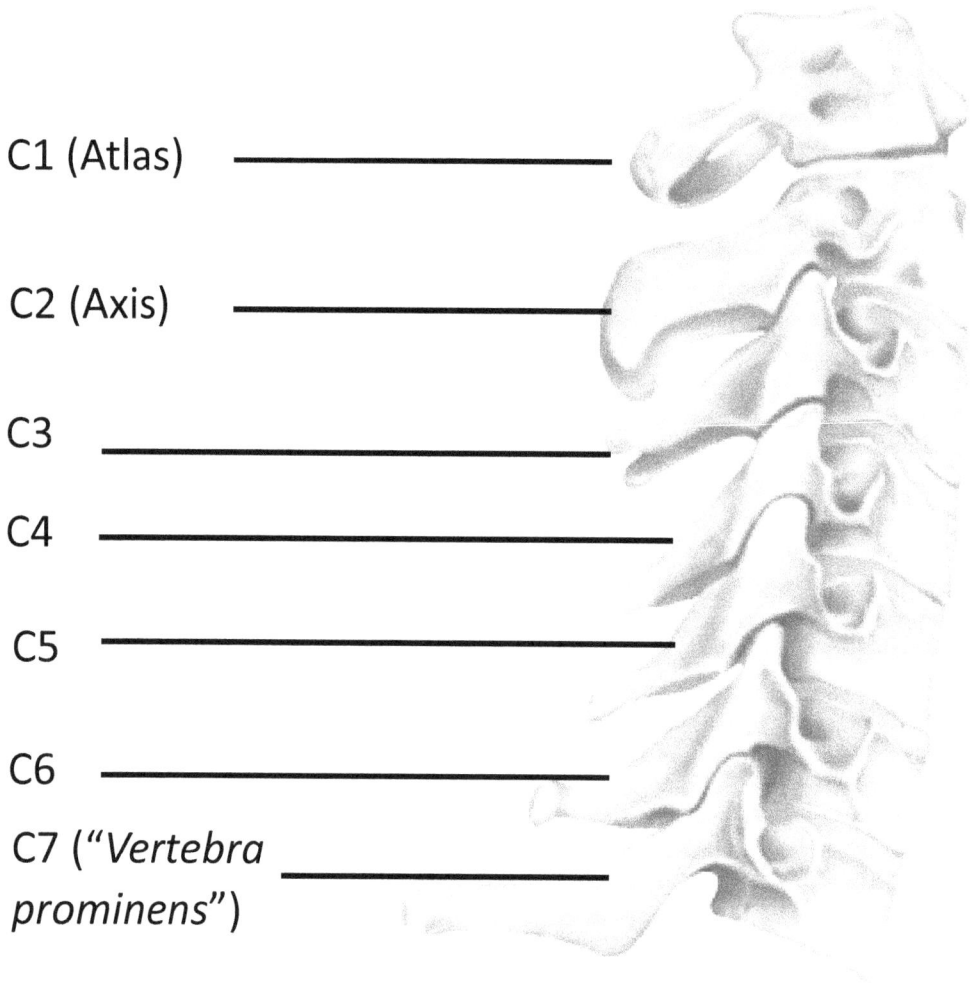

There are many technics presented here and are arranged in order of simplicity and ease of learning.  Simply put, the earlier maneuvers can be utilized with little practice, and the more advanced ones can be mastered as one gains experience and develops the "touch".

## ASSESSMENT

### Examination of the Cervical Spine

60°    50°

45°    45°

80°    80°

First evaluate gross range of motion in three planes. Ask the patient to touch chin to chest, then to tilt the head as far back as possible.  Observe from the side and make note of the angles in both directions.   Flexion should be 50º; extension should be 60º.

Next observe from the front and ask the patient to try to touch each ear to the shoulder.   Lateral flexion should be 45º in both directions.

Now ask the patient to turn the head as far as possible to the side in both directions.  Ideal ROM should be 80º; but as little as 50º is still functional.  Make note of any difference from side to side.

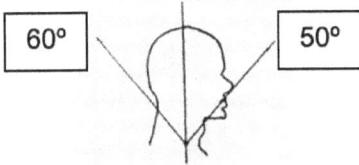

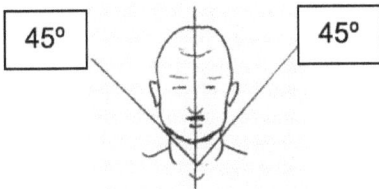

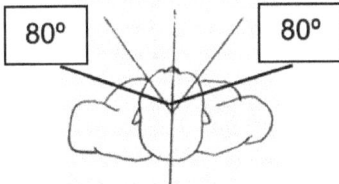

### Evaluating Cervical Curve

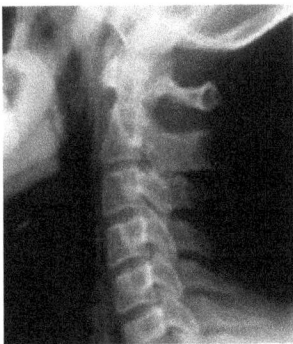

Normal

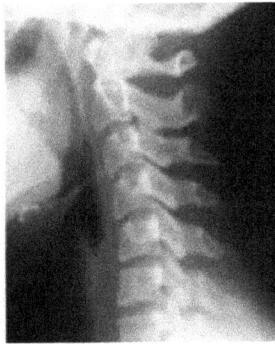

Reverse curve

Now palpate the cervical spine with the patient standing and facing forward.    Make contact with each spinous process and determine if the normal cervical lordosis is present.  Make note if the spine is unusually straight and/or the paracervical muscles are tight or rigid, or if there are any particularly tender points found.

**Evaluating Cervical Vertebral Restrictions**

1. With the patient supine, cradle the patient's head and palpate each set of transverse processes in turn while gently side bending the neck at that level. Make note of whether the vertebra feels the same at the end of the range of motion on each side. Your fingers should tell you if the vertebra moves farther to one side than to the other. Perform this with the patient's neck in flexion, then check again in extension. Move to the next vertebra and repeat.

2. Still cradling the head, let the fingers make contact under the occipital ridge and apply anterior-posterior movement to the cranium, to assess the amount of glide in the occipitoatlatal (OA) junction. Note any resistance to free movement. Then move to the succeeding vertebrae. See below.

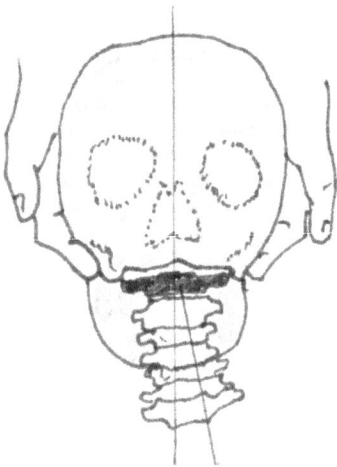

OA junction restricted on right

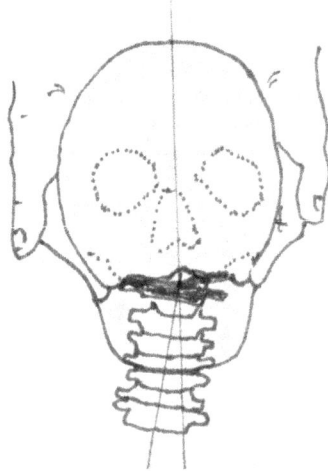

OA junction unrestricted on left

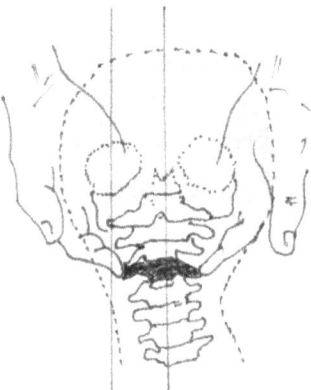

C3 normal ROM on right

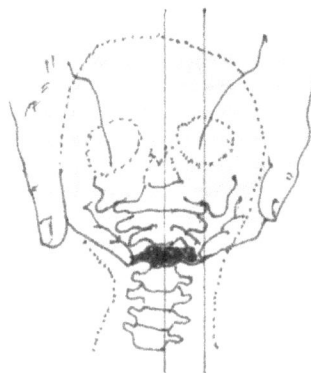

C3 ROM restricted on left

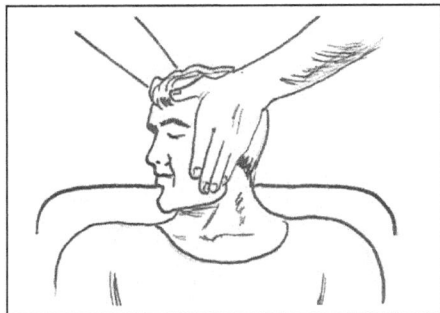

3. With the patient's neck in full flexion, rotate the head fully to one side and the other, evaluating range of motion in the axis. Compare the feel of one side to the other as well as the degree of passive motion. If the end feel of the motion is different, or the degree of rotation is reduced, it is positive for a C1-C2 restriction.

Note: Any sensation of excess play in the cervical spine indicates ligamentous laxity and mobilization with impulse is contraindicated.

**Cervical Compression Test (Spurling's maneuver)**

In cases where there is radiculopathy, there is a question of whether the source is a cervical disc or whether it may be thoracic outlet syndrome.

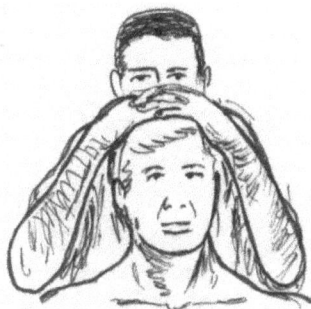

Place hands on the patient's crown, as in the illustration. Apply downward pressure and ask patient if this elicits pain. This is used to detect cervical or brachial plexus nerve compression by increasing the compression momentarily. Pain down the arm indicates nerve root compression, but not thoracic outlet syndrome. Although not an absolute indicator, it can be used to differentiate pain in the region that may or may not be due to nerve compression.

**Cervical Compression Test (Spurling's maneuver)**

**To differentiate simple neck stiffness from meningitis:**

In meningitis, resistance and pain is present when the neck is flexed forward but not when rotated. A stiff neck is painful when the head is pointed down and turned.
Brudzinski's sign #1: Flexing the neck produces flexure movements in both legs.
Brudzinski's sign #2: Maximally flexing the knee and hip joints of one leg produces flexure movements in the other leg.

## When vertebral fracture is suspected:

The Soto-Hall test is primarily used when fracture of a vertebra is suspected. The patient lies supine without pillows. One hand of the examiner is placed on the sternum of the patient, using a mild pressure to prevent either lumbar or thoracic flexion. The other hand of the examiner is cradled under the patient's occiput, and the head is slowly flexed toward the chest. Flexion of the head and neck toward the chest progressively creates a pull on the posterior spinal ligaments. When the spinous process of the injured vertebra is reached, acute local pain is experienced by the patient.

## Pre-screen all patients for vascular risk:
Extend and rotate the neck, and if vertigo or any sensory disturbance occurs (visual or auditory), do not use mobilization with impulse.

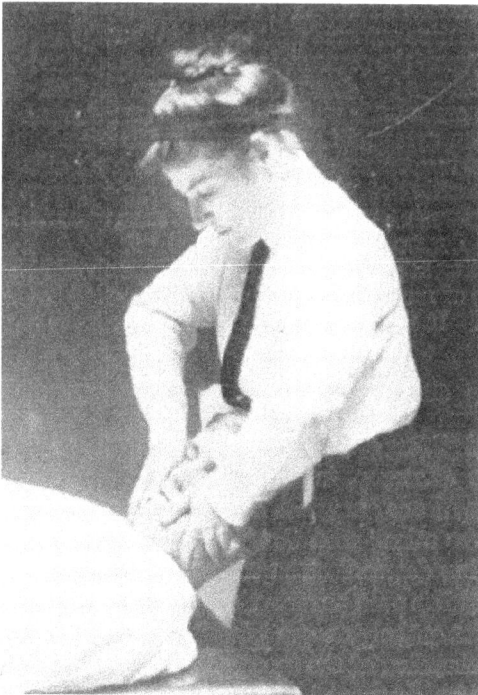

Neck in **flexion** before mobilization, as illustrated in *Osteopathic Mechanics*, by Ashmore

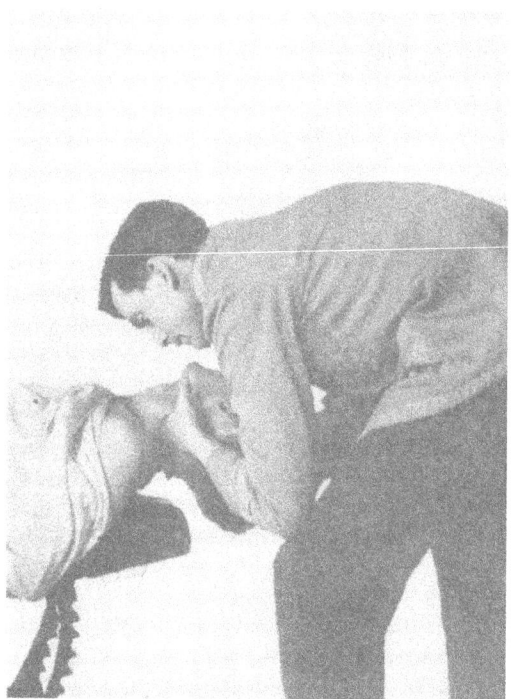

Neck in **extension** before mobilization, as illustrated in *Chiropractic Technic and Practice*, by Loban. The Posterior Cervical Move, as it is called, is not recommended.

# MOBILIZATION WITHOUT IMPULSE

The cervical spine is the most in need of preliminary treatment, due to the propensity of the paracervical muscles to tighten in response to anxiety or discomfort. Massage, mechanical vibration, guided passive range of motion, PNF, and most importantly, *verbally assuring* the patient will go a long way in preparing the body for a cervical maneuver. The neck should be treated methodically and unhurriedly, and if the patient is still tense in the cervicobrachial region, it is best not to use any mobilization with impulse.

## PNF

1. Locate the major muscle involved in the restriction of motion after assessing the range of motion in all three planes.
2. Relax and lengthen those muscles by stretching the patient's neck in the direction of restriction.
3. When the barrier is reached, ask the patient to try to move the head back against the resistance of your hand. This isometric contraction should last about seven seconds.
4. Tell the patient to relax the tension, breathe in, and breathe out. When the patient breathes out, use the anchoring hand to again guide the head toward the restriction. The second stretch should go farther than the first. If the normal range of motion is not achieved, repeat the process two more times.

## PROM
### Supine Traction with Circumduction

Site of restriction: Anywhere in the cervical spine, particularly if there is disc protrusion.

Patient position: Supine, with large bolster under the knees to prevent sliding. Head is extended off the table.

Technic:
1. Stand at the head of the table, with feet positioned ideally so as to prevent the table legs from being pulled back during the procedure.
2. One hand cups the chin and creates traction on the spine.
3. The other hand grasps the occiput and both supports the head and pulling to aid in creating traction.
4. Perform slow rotary motions, tracing a vertical circle with the head. The motions should not come close to the full range of motion. Maintain traction throughout.

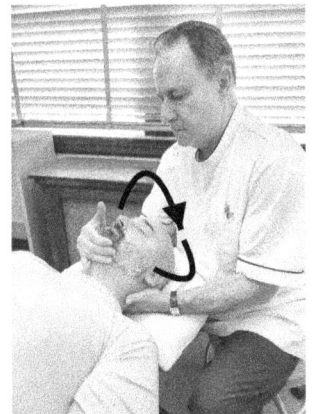

5.  Make 6-7 circumductions and slowly relax the traction.
6.  Ask patient to sit up and move the head in all directions to assess the results of the maneuver.  If there is no increase in range of motion, repeat the maneuver. It is permissible to perform several times before ending the session.
    * If there is strong pain, discontinue immediately.
    * There is typically crepitation in the cervical spine heard by the patient, and this should be explained in order to allay fears.

### Supine Rotation with Springing

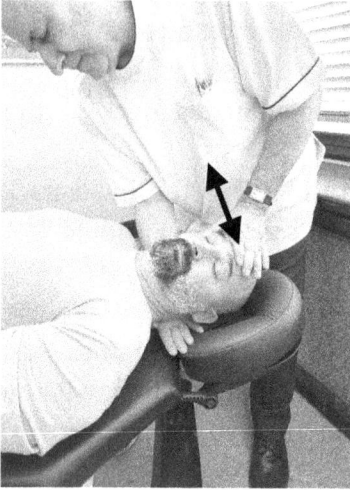

Site of restriction:  Upper cervical spine

Patient position:  Supine
Technic:
1. Operator stands at the side of the table.  Rotate the patient's head to the left, insert the thenar eminence of your hand below the mastoid process of the patient's left side.
2. The other hand is placed on the temporal bone and a gentle springing pressure is made downward toward the table.    After a few mobilizations, switch sides, approaching from the opposite side of the table.

### Supine Rotation with Fulcrum

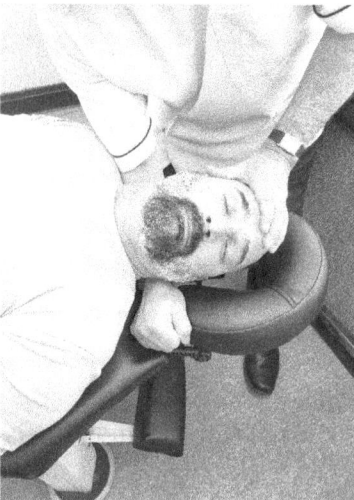

Site of restriction:  Upper cervical spine

Patient position:  Supine
Technic:
1. Operator stands at the side of the table.  Insert your right forearm under the cervical spine parallel with the shoulders.  The hand rests on the side of the table.
2. Patient's head is rotated left by gentle guided pressure on the temporal bone by the other hand.
3. Roll the head from neutral to rotation several times, then switch sides.   Considerable pressure is possible with a firm fulcrum such as this, so be extremely gentle with the anchoring hand.

# CERVICAL #1

**The "Lake Recoil" Upper Cervical Maneuver**

Site of restriction:  Atlantooccipital joint

Patient position:  Seated upright.

Technic:

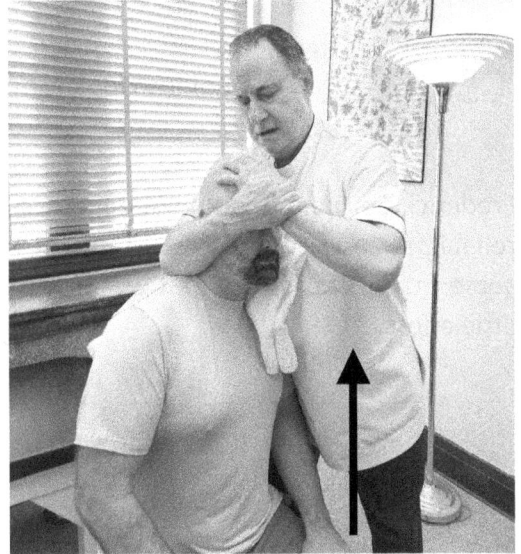

1. Seat the patient on a medium to low height stool.
2. Stand on the left of the patient, and put patient's left arm behind him.
3. The left hand of the doctor is then placed on the forehead of the patient with the heel of the hand on the frontal ridge of the nose, while the fingers rest lightly on the forehead.  No pressure should be exerted.  The right arm encircles the head all around.  You may be able to let the fingers rest lightly on the wrist of the left hand.  The stabilizing contact is made just over the occiput, lambdoidal sutures, and the mastoid bones; and in order for the fleshy part of the forearm to fit snugly on the skull, turn the head to the left three times very slowly, then bring head to dead center.  To make sure it is in dead center, bend the head forward a little, then bring it back. Now put your feet in position for a proper body balance, so you will not slip.
4. Bend the knees.
5. Next bring your chest over against the patient's head, padding the contact with a folded towel between his head and your chest.  Now stretch the head of the patient upward slightly until all slack is taken out, while instructing the patient to inhale and exhale.  When the breath is almost completely expelled, give a quick upward thrust by straightening the knees, which may slightly raise the patient off the stool.  The pressure used is less than fifty pounds.  There will be a distinct "click" sensation to the patient from the realignment of the atlas.
6. Repeat on the right side, reversing the position of the arms.

31

The amount of pull applied in the preliminary movement (removing the slack) ranges between 5 to l0 pounds. The amount of pull in the upward "jerk" is between 20 to 25 pounds.  It is Important to note that the human neck can endure pulls up to several hundred pounds.  This is a very safe maneuver.

- Do not hurry; make positive contacts first.
- Do not let the encircling arm slip.
- Do not press hard on the forehead.
- Watch that the ear is not squeezed by the encircling arm.

# CERVICAL #2   Collins Hook Maneuver

Frederick Collins taught a maneuver that he called the "Hook Move", which he felt was reliable for a variety of restrictions of the Occipitoatlantal (OA) joint.   While it takes some practice, it stands out as a surprisingly gentle and painless maneuver requiring little effort.

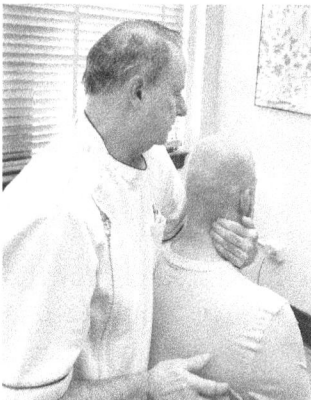

Site of restriction:    Atlantoaxial joint (C1-2) lateral malposition

Patient position:  Seated upright.

Technic:

To illustrate, we will assume that there is a right lateral displacement of the Atlas.   Simply reverse the description for a left side restriction.   The procedure follows:

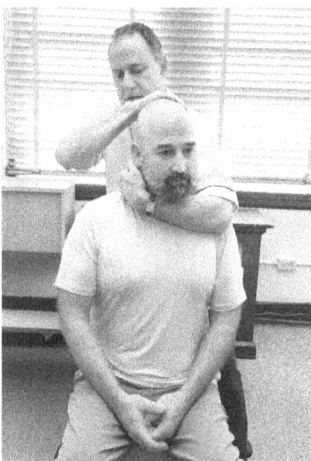

1. Stand behind the patient.   Reach over the patient's left shoulder and place your left elbow against the anterior shoulder (or pectorals, depending on the size differential between the two parties), reaching with the hand to the opposite side of patient's neck.
2. Make firm contact on the right transverse process of the axis with the palmar side of the distal phalanx of the middle finger of your left hand.   The forearm is parallel with the shoulders.  This is the mobilizing hand.
3. Reach with the right hand behind the patient's head across to the left side of the head above the ear, with the fingers flexed just enough for steady contact.   This is the

anchoring hand.

4. Using the right hand to side bend the patient's head to the right, feel for the barrier.

5. Holding that position for a moment, now <u>simultaneously</u>:

   - Pull the head with the right hand to create side bending to the right beyond the restrictive barrier
   - Apply impulse with the middle finger against the transverse process, and
   - Use your left elbow to make a snappy movement that pushes the patient's left shoulder posteriorly.

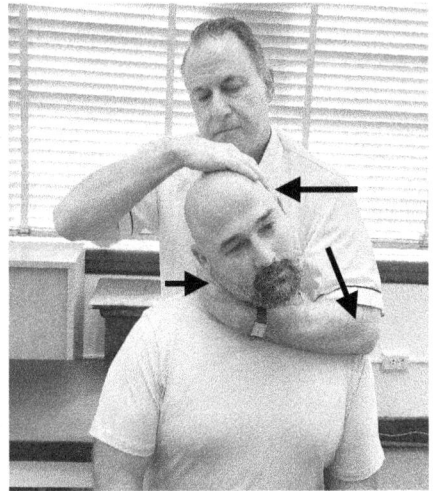

If you decisively make these movements simultaneously, the correction of the restriction will be effortless and there is no sensation of strain on the part of the patient. Collins said "It does not require force...it is having a perfect contact and a unique spontaneity of thrust."

# CERVICAL #3   Seated Cervical Rotary Maneuver

Site of restriction: C2-C7
Patient position: Seated upright, slightly slumped.

Technic:

1. Have patient seated on a stool with the head flexed forward (not a chair with a back). Stand to the side perpendicularly with feet apart and bend the knees until your sternum is level with the patient's ear. Make sure the neck is relatively relaxed. Do not mobilize unless you are able to get the patient to relax. The more relaxed, the less force is necessary to achieve mobilization.

2. Ask him to touch his chin to his chest and turn the head toward you as far as he can.

3. Position the palm of the contact hand over the angle of the mandible, with the thumb extending to the temporal area and the fingers wrapping around the neck (making an "L" shape), as in the illustration. The finger pads contact the transverse processes and press

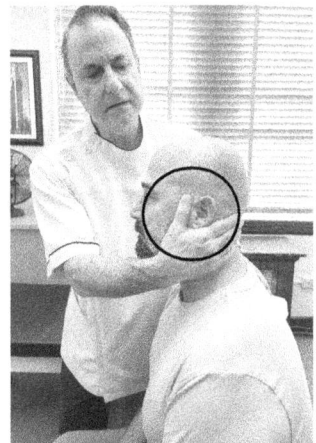

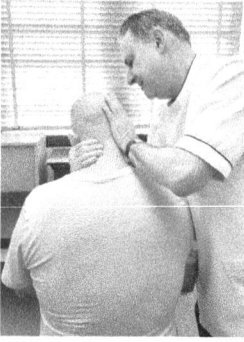

firmly. Your wrist and forearm will be aligned with the mandible. Elbow should point down.

4. Anchoring hand is now placed in the similar position on the other side, but no pressure is placed on the transverse processes.

5. When the barrier is felt, do not allow the head to rotate away even slightly. Now an impulse is made by rotating the head further, quickly. The far hand makes the impulse, and the other hand supports and guides the motion.

6. Treat the other side by the same procedure, mirror image.

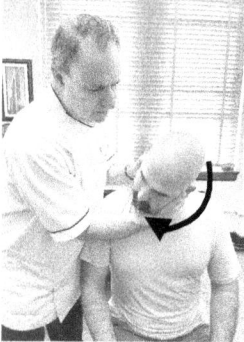

- There should be no pressure on the chin or jaw.
- While this is practically a universal cervical mobilization for all vertebrae from C2 to possibly C7, you can include C1 by simply placing the index finger firmly under the occiput. Otherwise, the index finger is positioned over the transverse process of C2.
- If range of motion evaluation reveals a restriction in rotation, you can mobilize the axis by applying pressure to C2 only with no pressure on any of the lower vertebrae.
- More pressure can be exerted by the finger pad on the target vertebra (eg., C3, C4) to isolate it.
- It is usually good to mobilize both sides.

# CERVICAL #4   Cervical Rotary Maneuver, supine

Site of restriction:  C2-C7

Patient position:  Supine.

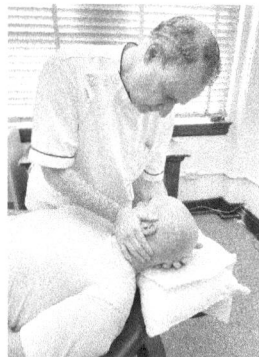

Some people will relax more when reclining, so use this maneuver if Cervical #3 is not successful.

Technic:

1. Stand to the side of the table. Bend your knees, leaning forward and toward the head of the table.

2. Anchoring hand raises the head above the table and in the same position as the vertical version. Contact hand reaches to the opposite side and makes firm contact with the fingers on the transverse processes.

3. Rotate head toward you until you reach the barrier, hold for a moment to assess relaxation, and if relaxed, apply impulse in the form of further rotation with a snappy movement.

4. Change your position to the other side of the table to mobilize the other side.

# CERVICAL #5　Atlantooccipital Maneuver, supine

Site of restriction:  AO joint, C1

Patient position:  Supine.

Technic:
1. Operator stands at the side of the table on the side of restriction.  Cup the patient's chin in your far hand, letting the head rest on your forearm.  This is the anchoring hand.
2. Index finger of the close hand (contact hand) is placed posterolateral to the posterior arch of the atlas.   The thumb extends naturally over the angle of the mandible.
3. The neck is flexed (see circle) and the head is side bent toward the site of restriction.
4. The head is rotated away from the site of restriction, and when the barrier is reached, impulse is delivered by a thrusting motion with the index finger toward the contralateral eye.

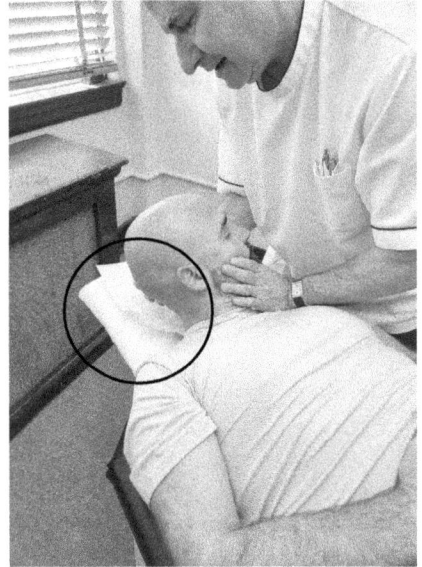

# CERVICAL #6   **Atlantoaxial Maneuver, supine**

Site of restriction:  C1, C2

Patient position:  Supine.

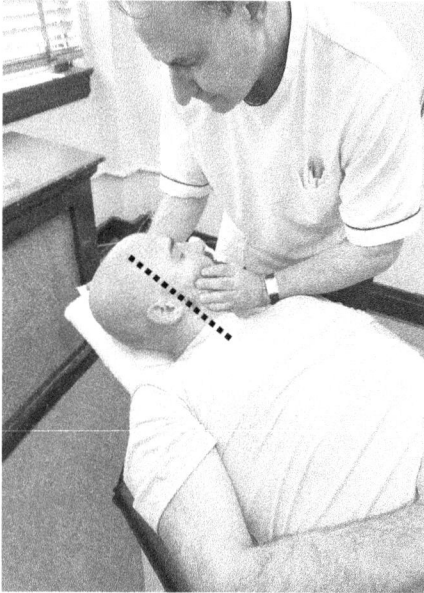

Technic:

1. Operator stands at the side of the table on the side of restriction.  With the chin cupped and the head supported by the forearm, position the index finger against the posterior arch of the atlas (C1) or the axis (C2), as the case may be.   The thumb falls over the angle of the mandible in either case.

2. Slightly side bend the head in the direction of the restriction.  The cervical spine is **in a neutral position**, neither flexed nor extended (dotted line).

3. Rotate the head away from the side of restriction, and when the barrier is reached, apply impulse in a further rotation.  The index finger only immobilizes the transverse process.  It does not thrust in this maneuver.

# CERVICAL #7  Supine Lateral Maneuver with Impulse

Site of restriction:  C3-C6

Patient position:  Supine, with the head beyond the table surface.

Technic:
This is a maneuver for a laterally-displaced vertebra discovered by palpation.

1. Operator stands at the head of the table. To illustrate, we will say that C4 is laterally displaced to the left.
2. Take the patient's head in your right hand, grasping the occiput with the fingers and pressing the thenar eminence against the patient's temporal bone.  Hold the head with the cervical spine in a neutral position.
3. The left hand is used as a fulcrum.  The base of the index finger (MCP joint) is pressed against the C4 left transverse process with the fingertips against the clavicle for steadying.  Extend the thumb as much as possible to avoid the trachea.
4. At the moment of relaxation, strongly and quickly push both hands toward each other.  This forces the patient's head to the left and his neck to the right.

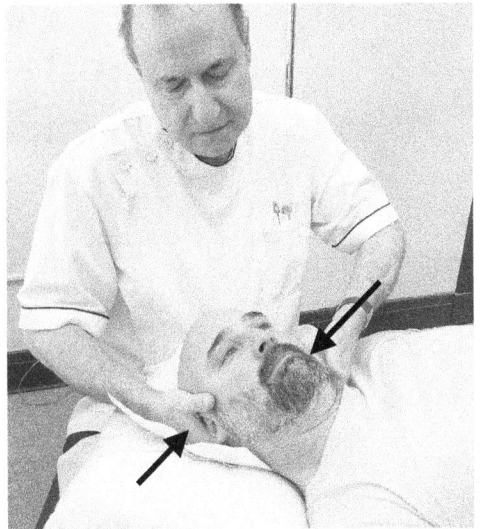

# CERVICAL #8    Supine Traction with Impulse

Site of restriction:  Anywhere in the cervical spine

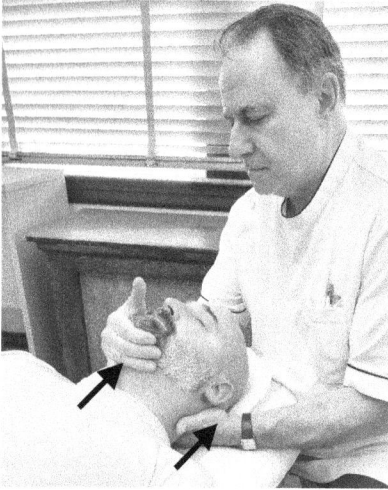

Patient position:  Supine.

Technic:
1.Stand at the head of the table.  Grasp the chin with one hand and the occiput with the other.
2.Apply traction to the spine, gradually and gently.
3.At the end point of the traction, suddenly pull with both hands, simultaneously lifting the head off the table slightly.
•This is a general corrective maneuver, as a particular restriction tends to release when traction plus impulse is applied.

# CERVICAL #9    Supine Anteroposterior Gliding Maneuver

Technically, this is not a mobilization with impulse, but it is of value when any of the foregoing maneuvers have failed to resolve the cervical restriction.  Consider this as a "back up plan".

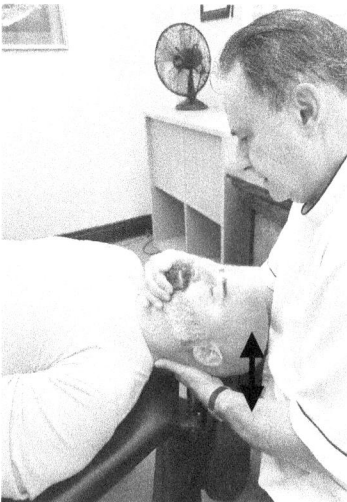

Site of restriction:  Any cervical vertebra

Patient position:  Supine with head extended off the head of the table, large bolster under the knees to prevent sliding.

Technic:
Because this maneuver places a strain on the upper lip, it is necessary to place a pad (foam or rolled up toweling) between your contact hand and the patient's mouth.
1. Place one of your legs against the table to prevent sliding.
2. Place one hand under the occiput, supporting the head and applying traction.

38

(cont.)
3. Place the other hand, with padding in place over the mouth.
4. While maintaining traction and neutral position of the spine with the lower hand, use the top hand to apply strong pressure downward over the mouth. This induces an anterior-posterior gliding of the cervical vertebrae. Hold for a few seconds, then release the downward pressure without easing up on the traction force.
5. Repeat a few times, then have the patient sit up and assess.

# CERVICAL #10 Supine Lateral Gliding Maneuver

Once again, this is not a mobilization with impulse. When mobilization with impulse has failed to resolve the cervical restriction, this maneuver, as well as Cervical #9, can reduce the displacement without force.

Site of restriction: Any cervical vertebra

Patient position: Supine with head extended off the head of the table, large bolster under the knees to prevent sliding. If an assistant is present, it is advantageous to have the assistant stand to the side and grasp the far arm, pressing the patient's near arm against his sides.

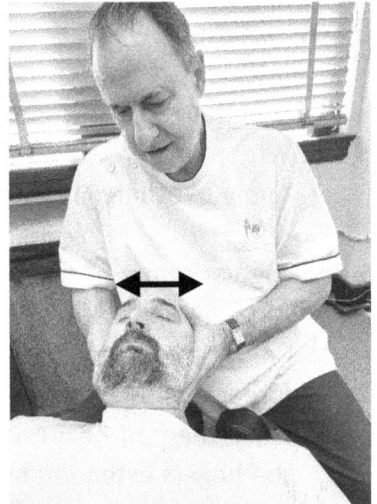

Technic: Explain the procedure to the patient to allay any apprehension. The maneuver is painless.
1. Support the head with both hands. The thenar eminences apply an alternating pressure to the temporal bones while the thumbs maintain the alignment of the head to prevent any side bending.
2. Slowly press laterally in one direction and then the other, alternating for several minutes.

# CERVICAL #11   Prone Lower Cervical Rotation

This maneuver frees the cervicothoracic junction.

Site of restriction:  C7-T1

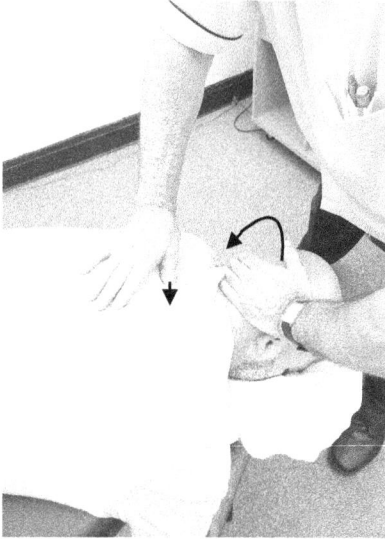

Patient position:  Prone

Technic:
1. Operator stands at the side of the table; In this example, the left side.
2. Locate the spinous process of T1.  Gently but firmly press the pad of the right thumb against the SP of T1, with the web of the hand resting on the trapezius.
3. Place your left hand on the patient's temporal bone with your forearm as parallel as possible with the edge of the table.
4. Ask patient to inhale and slowly exhale.
5. As the patient begins exhaling, induce a side bending force through T1 with the right hand while simultaneously rotating the head to reach the restrictive barrier.
6. When the barrier is reached, impulse is applied with both hands.
7. Apply to other side by reversing directions.

## Side-lying Variation:
1. Face the right side-lying patient from the side of the table.
2. Cradle the patient's head with your left hand, supporting the weight with the forearm and resting the fingers over the occiput.
3. Place the pad of the right thumb against the left transverse process of T1, with the fingers extended back over the trapezius.
4. As patient to inhale and slowly exhale.  As he exhales, begin to take up "slack" as usual, gently raising patient's head.  It is helpful to bend your rear knee to engage your body in directing pressure through your thumb.
5. When you have engaged the barrier, deliver an impulse to the transverse process while simultaneously making a counter force with the anchoring hand.
Note:  The anchoring hand may need to create some flexion or extension in order to engage the restriction.

# CERVICAL #12 **Prone Cervicothoracic Maneuver**

This maneuver frees the cervicothoracic junction.

Site of restriction:  C7-T1

Patient position:  Prone

Technic:
1. Operator stands at the head of the table, knees bent but spine straight and bending forward from the hips.  Your lead leg should be in contact with the table.
2. Place web of your hand against the superior angle of the contralateral scapula.
3. The other hand makes contact with the patient's temporal bone.  The forearm must be parallel to the head of the table or shoulder line.
4. Ask patient to inhale and slowly exhale.
5. As patient begins exhaling, gradually take up the "slack" in the tissues and engage the barrier.
6. With the forearm directly in line with the hand, direct an oblique force through the scapula in the direction of the axilla, while simultaneously the other hand creates a rotational force to the patient's right.  Equal force is generated by each hand.
7. Reverse positions to treat the other side if needed.

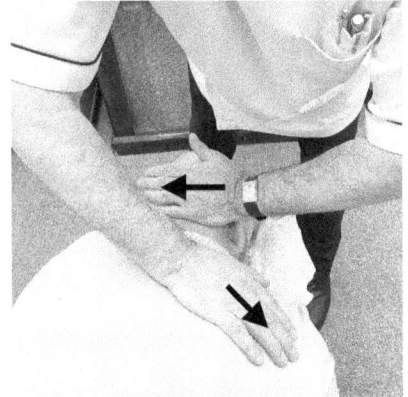

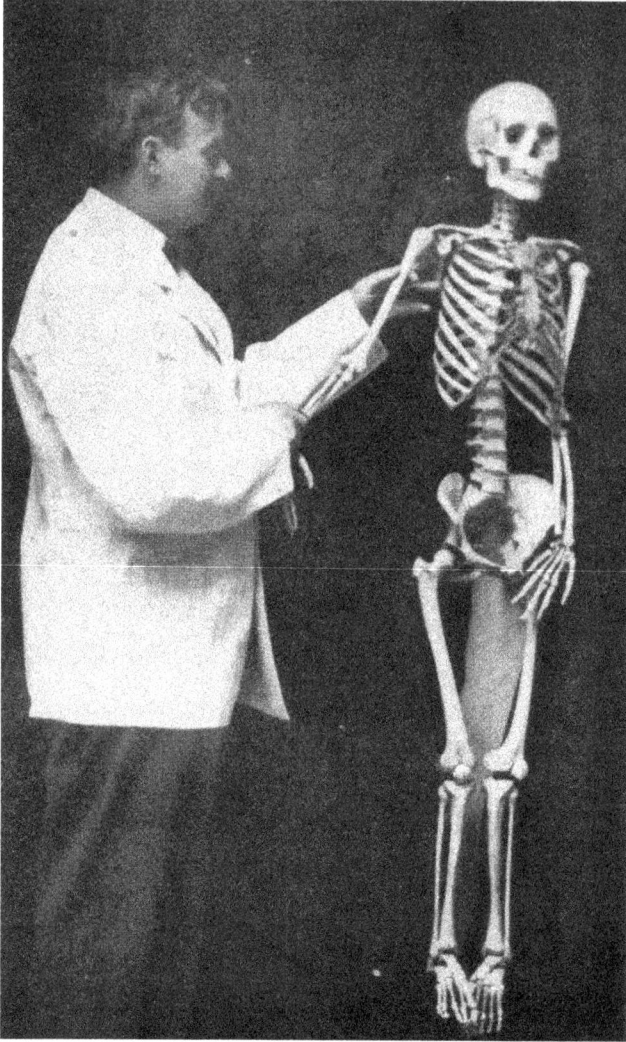

Dr. Frederick Collins and his teaching assistant, at
First National University of Naturopathy, 1924

# SECTION FOUR

## THORACIC MANEUVERS

---

## ASSESSMENT

---

Inspection, percussion and palpation are the major methods for examining the spine. Adjunct methods include thermographic measurement, electrical skin resistance measurement, and dolorimetric readings (applying standardized pressure to see where there is tenderness). Imaging ranges from X-rays and MRIs to contour analysis and thermograms.

Of all these, palpation is the most important. The position of the patient must be changed accordingly as the examiner checks for different types of abnormalities. For example, lateral curvatures are best detected when the patient is bending forward, often while sitting. Rigidity of the spinal column, thickening of the spinal ligaments, degree of separation of the spinous processes—all are better detected with the patient in a lateral recumbent position. Other postural abnormalities are spotted more easily when the patient is standing normally.

The back must be bare for the examination. Have the patient standing first, and make note of any postural deviations from the norm. Remember that an unnatural posture may have become "natural" to him or her by virtue of the pathology. Attempts to "normalize" the posture during the exam will obscure the true state. The examiner should make every attempt to observe the patient's habitual posture and gait.

**1. Observe the patient from the rear.** Make note of any deviation from the normal level in:
- The horizontal line of the shoulders
- The inferior angles of the scapulae
- The iliac crests

Careful inspection often uncovers asymmetry of the waistline and hips. For example, a deeper cut to the waist on one side, typically accompanied by a higher or larger contour of the hip on the same side, is an indicator of torsion of the spine.

**2. Now observe the patient from the side** and note any exaggerated or flattened thoracic curve, and also any exaggerated or flattened lumbar curve as well. The ears should hang over or slightly in front of the shoulder in good posture. More forward positioning of the head, as indicated by the vertical alignment of the ears, can indicate problems with the thoracic spine.

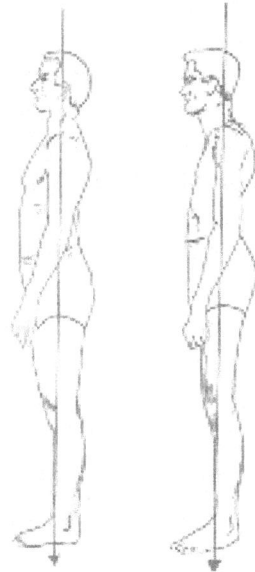

When a person stands erect, a mechanically correct posture causes the various segments of the body to be placed so that each supports the one immediately above it, against the action of gravity. These segments will make a straight vertical line, which is considered the long axis of the body. Authorities differ as to the exact location of this line, but the illustration here is fairly reliable. Seen in profile, the attachment of the ear, acromion, the iliac crest, and a point just anterior to the Calcaneus will ideally form a vertical line. With imperfect posture, a zigzag shape is seen.

Also note any uneven muscular development, changes in coloring, rashes, skin growths, injected blood vessels, scars or evidence of surgical operations, etc.

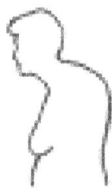 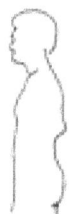

An exaggerated thoracic curve is *kyphosis*.

A sudden alteration in the thoracic curvature is called *angular kyphosis*. The unusually prominent spinous process found there is called a *gibbus*.

Kyphosis        Gibbus

**3.    Now have the patient sit in a slightly bent-forward position**, hands on knees or arms loosely folded.    Stand behind the patient and use the thumb or index finger to perform a friction against the skin, rubbing down the spine taking care to only contact the tips of the spinous processes. This is in order to make the skin red.    Observe if the red line so created has a true plumb or vertical orientation. Make note if there is any deviation from the midline.

Now make contact with each individual spinous process, pressing with the pad of the index finger.    During this process, pay attention to whether any of the spinous processes feel abnormally displaced anteriorly or posteriorly.    Usually a vertebra that has moved anteriorly will be very tender to palpation.    Make note of which vertebra is in such condition.

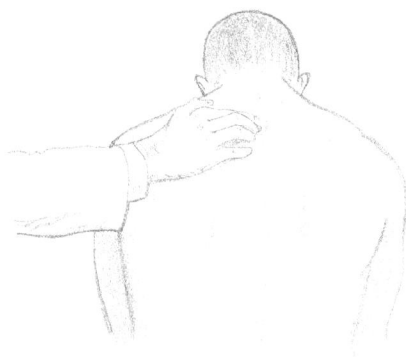

If the spacing between any of the vertebrae seems unusually wide or narrow, press between them with the tip of the index finger to assess the separation or approximation of the pair of spinous processes.

**4.    Now pass the index and middle fingers down opposite sides of the spinal column**, paying attention to several things:

1.    Watch for lateral deviations of the vertebrae.
        There is often tenderness in the tissues on the convex side of the deviation.
2.    In any individual vertebra that seems deviated laterally, palpate the transverse processes to determine if they are truly laterally displaced, or if there is just a bent spinous process.
3.    Watch for lateral swerving of whole regions of the spine, indicating scoliosis.

4. Note any exaggerations or lessening of the normal curvature of the spine. A flattening of the spine between the shoulder blades is the most common abnormality. Exaggerated curve (*kyphosis*) is also common.

If lateral curvature (*scoliosis*) has been detected, check with patient standing forward bending with feet together. Allow the arms to hang down. One will typically see asymmetrical muscular contour in the back with lateral curvatures, when the subject is bending over and the thoracic spine is viewed from the rear.
Make note of:

- Rib cage elevation on one side
- Prominent unilateral lumbar region musculature.
- Pronated foot, if present.
- Inequalities in leg length.

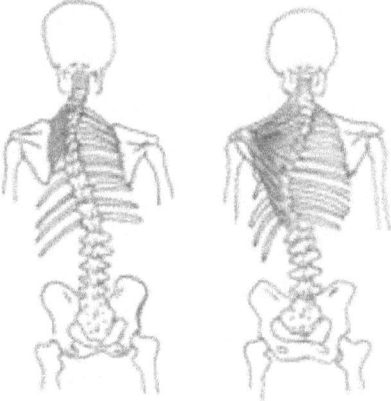

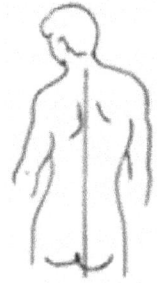

Scoliosis

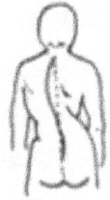

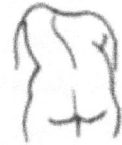

A quick examination can also be made from in front of the patient (same forward bending position), assessing rib cage elevation visually. This is known as Adam's test.

There may be one curvature (C curve), or there may be two (S curve). In the latter case, the spine compensates for the first curve by deviating to the other side. Individuals over the age of eleven with lateral curvature should be referred for X-rays.

Note: If a lateral curve is seen on standing but it disappears on forward bending or lateral recumbent position, the scoliosis is functional (also called postural), not structural; it should respond quickly to well-chosen treatment. Structural scoliosis is defined as being caused by malformations of the vertebrae.

Radiographic imaging by X-ray is the standard for quantifying curvatures that are more than 7 degrees deviant on palpatory and visual exam. This translates to a 20-degree deviation on X-ray, using Cobb's Angle, a method of identifying the uppermost and bottom vertebrae in the curve, drawing lines along the inferior borders to the point where they meet, and calculating the angle of deviation.

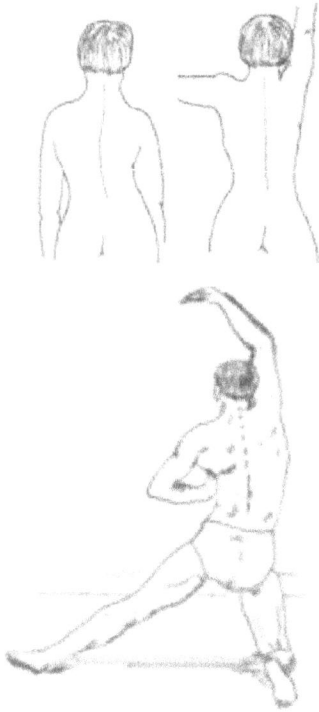

Key note position

Exercises that involve lateral bending toward the convex side are used to reduce functional scoliosis. The use of a "key-note" position can correct flexible cases. This is a device to allow the patient's spine to assume the correct position. For example, when the patient attempts to stand straight and presents a thoracic convex curve to the left, raising the arm to a certain height can bring into play muscles that will straighten the spine. In some cases, raising both arms, but to different positions, will achieve the correction.

Curvatures lower in the spine may require abduction of one leg, or everting a foot. When the exact position is found that eliminates the curve, it is said to be the "key-note" position for the case. The patient is instructed to assume this position many times a day, and to do specialized exercises to strengthen the muscles that power that posture.

## SCOLIOSIS CHECKLIST

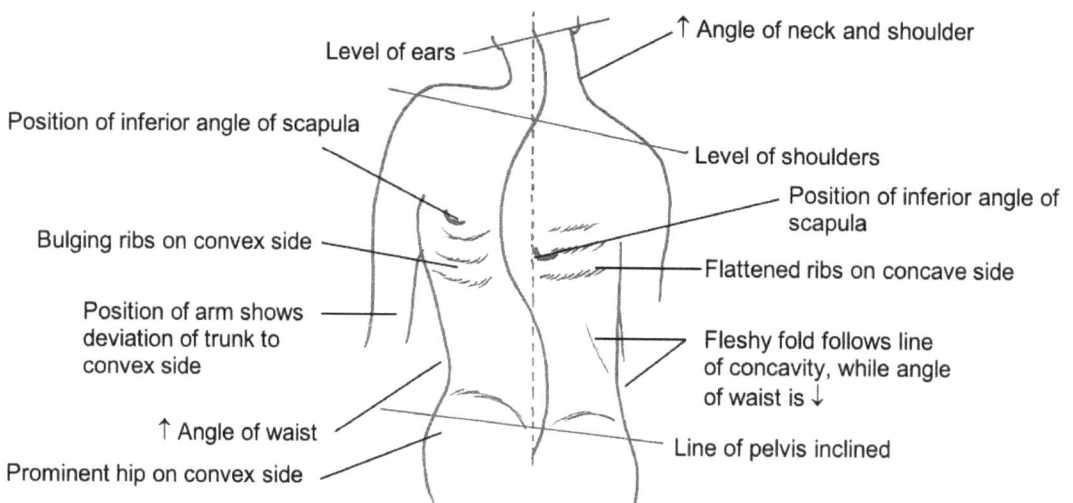

Level of ears

↑ Angle of neck and shoulder

Position of inferior angle of scapula

Level of shoulders

Position of inferior angle of scapula

Bulging ribs on convex side

Flattened ribs on concave side

Position of arm shows deviation of trunk to convex side

Fleshy fold follows line of concavity, while angle of waist is ↓

↑ Angle of waist

Line of pelvis inclined

Prominent hip on convex side

# MOBILIZATION WITHOUT IMPULSE

**PROM**

**Seated Traction Upper Thoracic**

1. Operator stands behind the seated patient with his foot on a stool and the knee acting as a stabilizing base for the arm.
2. The right hand grasps the occiput and the left hand grasps the forehead.
3. Traction on the upper thoracic spine is created by holding a firm grip on the head and gradually raising and lowering the

**Side Upper Thoracic Leverage**

1. Patient is side lying on the contralateral side from where the restriction is found. His upper arm is dropped down the thorax.
2. Operator sits on the edge of the table. Your right arm locks the patient's arm as you reach posteriorly and make a contact with the thumb against the lower of the two vertebrae that form the restriction. The left hand and forearm support the head in flexion.
3. Cupping the patient's head, draw slowly upward into a side bending position while maintaining pressure on the transverse process with the other hand. Lower the head and repeat a few times. One can also rotate the head a bit while side bending.

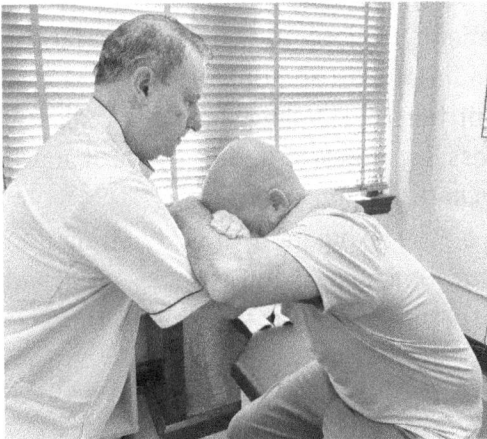

**Under-Over**

1. Have patient cross arms across chest with the thumbs hooked in the antecubital fossae..
2. Stand in front , place hands under the patient's arms and over his shoulders with your fingers making a firm contact with the transverse processes of the affected spinal segment.
3. Draw the patient toward you as you apply leverage upward on the forearms and downward pressure through the fingers. Apply in a springing motion several times.

# THORACIC #1   "Nelson" Thoracic Lift

Site of restriction:  Upper thoracic, T1-T4

Patient position:  Seated

Technic:

1. Operator stands behind the seated patient with knees bent.  Reaching under the patient's arms, he applies what in wrestling is called a "full Nelson". The fingers are interlaced behind patient's neck and the operator's body is against patient's back.

2. Ask the patient to look downward as far as possible and to breathe in and out.

3. When patient begins exhaling, lean back slightly and exert pressure upward under the axillae to create traction in the spine.

4. At the end of the exhalation, quickly straighten the knees and, leaning slightly back, create a snappy impulse that releases the upper thoracic segments.

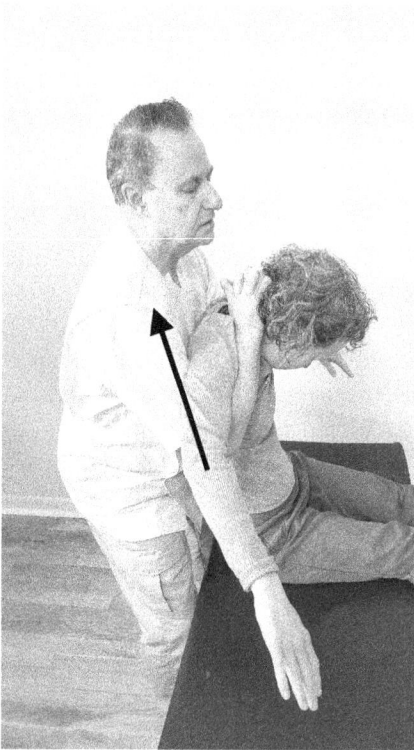

# THORACIC #2   Seated Thoracic Lift 1

Site of restriction:  Mid-thoracic, T4-T6 (as low as T12 in some cases)

Patient position:  Seated

Technic:
1. Operator behind seated patient. Patient is asked to clasp his fingers behind his neck.
2. Reach under the arms and take hold of patient's wrists.  Press your sternum against the lower site of restriction; i.e., the lower of the two vertebrae involved.
3. Patient is asked to breathe in and out.
4. At the end of exhalation, thrust your sternum forward while pulling back on the patient's arms.  This can also be done with the knee, covered with a cushion.

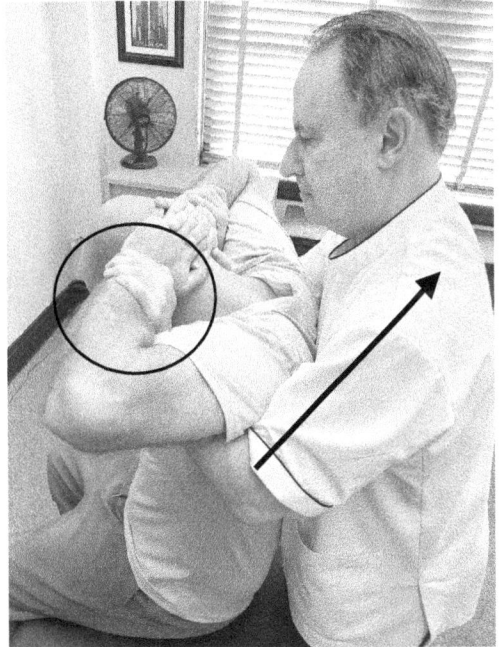

# THORACIC #3   Seated Thoracic Lift 2

Site of restriction:  Mid-thoracic, T4-T6 (as low as T12 in some cases)

Patient position:  Seated

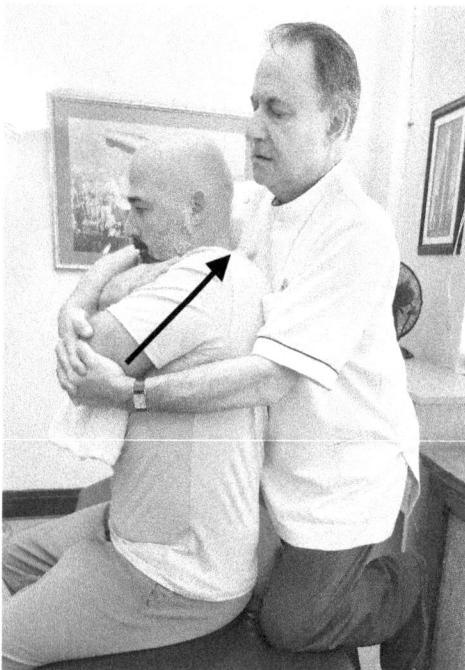

Technic:

1. Ask if there is any shoulder pathology.  If so, do not use.
2. Operator stands behind seated patient with knees bent.  Patient is asked to clasp his opposite shoulders and bring his elbows to his midline.  It is recommended that you place a rolled-up towel between his sternum and arms for cushioning.
3. Place a rolled-up towel between your chest and the lower of the two vertebrae that are restricted.
4. Reach around and grasp the patient's lower elbow, lacing your fingers for stability.
5. Ask patient to inhale and exhale.
6. Near the end of the exhalation, reduce the "slack" in the spine by leaning posteriorly and exerting a superior direction force on his arms
7. When you engage the barrier, straighten the knees and pull patient's arm to create the impulse.

# THORACIC #4   **Seated Thoracic Lift 3**

Site of restriction:  Lower thoracic, T9-T12

Patient position:  Seated

Technic:
1.  Operator stands behind patient. Patient is asked to place both hands on the back, overlapping.  Operator should position them so as to be over the restriction.

2. Pass your hands through the arms and around to the patient's chest and clasp the hands.  Your sternum (or abdomen, depending on height) should be pressed against the patient's hands (not done in this picture in order to show patient's arm position).

3. Ask patient to breathe in and out. During the exhale, lean back a bit and, at the end, quickly pull your arms backward toward your own chest, simultaneously thrusting forward with your own sternum.

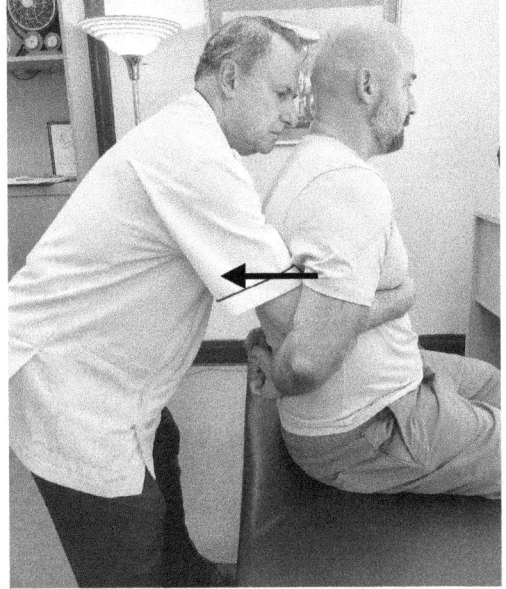

# THORACIC #5    **Seated Thoracic Lift #4**

Site of restriction:  Lower thoracic, T9-T12

Patient position:  Seated

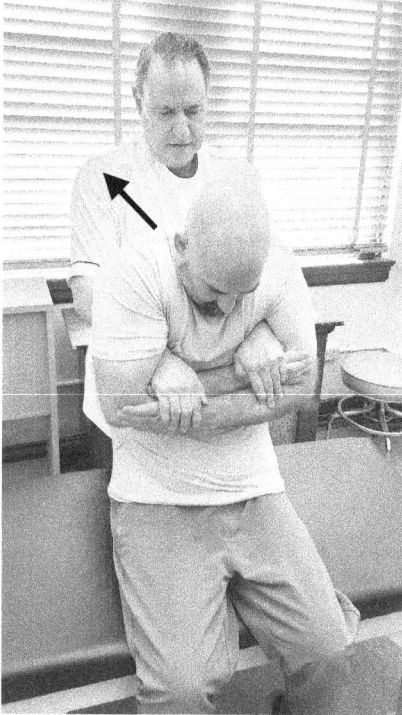

Technic:

1.Stand behind patient with knees flexed.  Patient is asked to grasp his elbows with his hands.

2.Slip your arms through his axillae and firmly grasp his forearms.

3.Press your sternum against his spine and ask him to breathe in and out.

4.As he exhales, pull him toward you and lean posteriorly, taking up the "slack".

5.At the end of the exhale, straighten your knees and quickly pull him further posteriorly and superiorly.

# THORACIC #6    **Facing Thoracic Maneuver**

Site of restriction:  T6-T12

Patient position:  Seated

Technic:
1.  Operator faces seated patient.  Patient is asked to clasp each hand on the opposite shoulder.
2. Lift patient's elbows and place them on your supraclavicular surfaces.
3. Reach around both sides of patient and make contact with the transverse processes of the lower of the two vertebrae in restriction.
4. Step backward, drawing patient toward you and extending his spine.  Instruct him to breathe in and out.
5. At the end of exhalation, apply impulse by suddenly pulling both hands simultaneously.

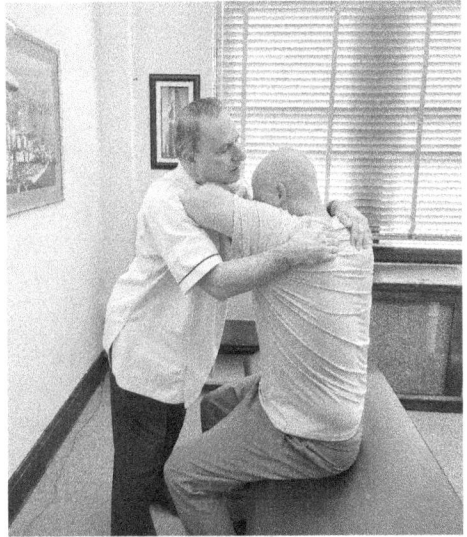

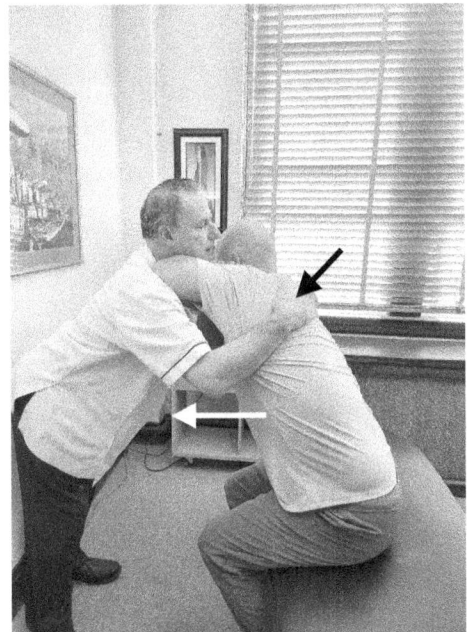

# THORACIC #7 Lower Thoracic Rotation Maneuver

Site of restriction: T8-T12

Patient position: Seated

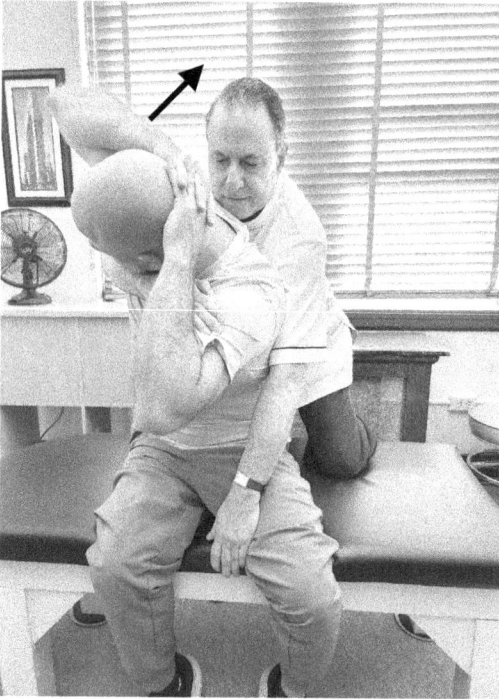

Technic:
1. Ask patient to clasp hands behind his neck.
2.Stand behind him and reach around to grasp patient's contralateral arm (his left arm with your right hand) and draw him around into rotation.
3.Reach with your other (left) hand between patient's legs and grasp the edge of the table, immobilizing the pelvis.
4.Produce rotation until the barrier is reached, then continue a bit farther while also pulling the back into extension, about 45 degrees.
5.Repeat on other side, reversing the grips.

This is a good maneuver for lower thoracic restrictions, and can be performed both with impulse and without impulse.

# THORACIC #8   **Prone Thoracic Thrust Maneuver**

Site of restriction:  T6-T11

Patient position:  Prone, or perpendicularly across table with head and arms hanging off.  There should be sufficient space for the chin so as to relax the cervicals.

Technic:
1.  Straddle patient with one knee on the table and other foot on the floor..
2. Place the hypothenar surfaces of both hands on the transverse processes of the vertebra to be released.
3. Ask patient to breathe in and out.
4. At the end of the exhale, deliver a thrust with both hands.   If the patient has a flexion restriction (reduced forward bending), apply the downward (P-A) thrust to the transverse processes of the lower of the two vertebrae in the restriction, in a caudal direction.  If there is an extension restriction (reduced back bending), apply the thrust to the transverse processes of the upper of the two vertebrae, and in a cephalic direction.  This will guide the facets in a flexion direction.

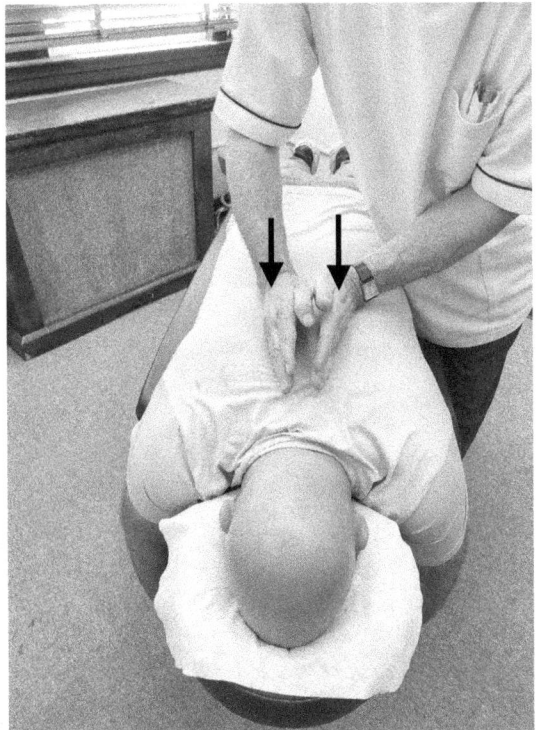

# THORACIC #9  Mid to Lower Thoracic Rotation Maneuver

This is a useful alternative when other thoracic maneuvers have failed.
Site of restriction:  T6-T11

Patient position:  Lateral recumbent.

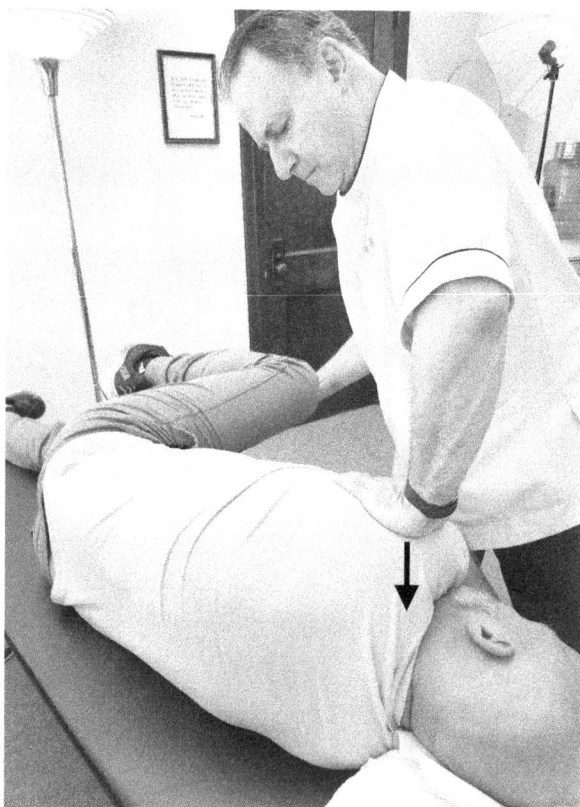

Technic:
1. Stand facing patient.
2. Flex patient's top hip and knee while the other leg remains in extension.
3. Place your cephalidad hand on the posterior aspect of the patient's shoulder and draw him into rotation.
4. Grasp patient's knee with your other hand and abduct the leg slightly.  This is the anchoring hand.
5. On the patient's exhale, thrust toward the table with the cephalidad hand, with the line of drive emanating from the hypothenar eminence or pisiform bone.

# RIBS

**First Rib Mobilization**

In this example, the restriction is on the left side.

Patient position: Supine

Technic:

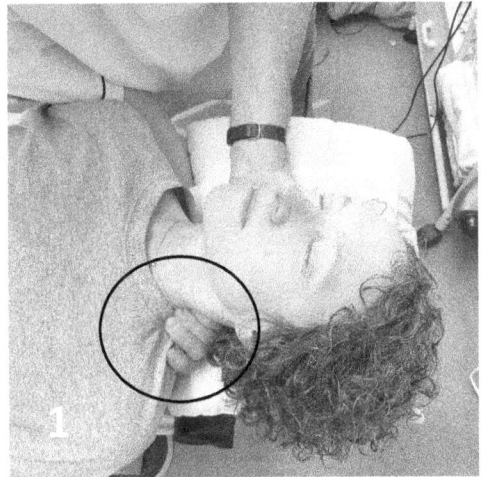

1. Stand on the right side of the table. Lift patient's right upper arm, allowing your right arm to pass under the back, so that your fingers can be placed over the left first rib.

2. Place your left hand under patient's right cervical region, with the fingers extending over the occiput. The thumb is in front of the ear extending toward the temporal bone.

3. Using the left hand, induce a slight flexion, left side bending, and right rotation until you feel you have locked the spine down to T1.

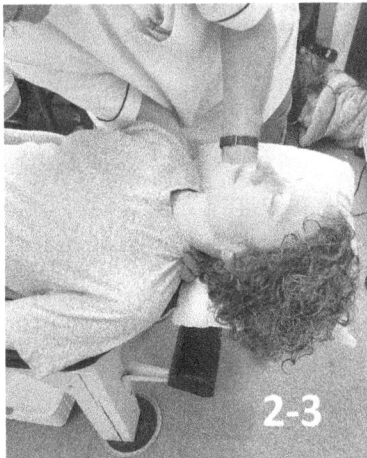

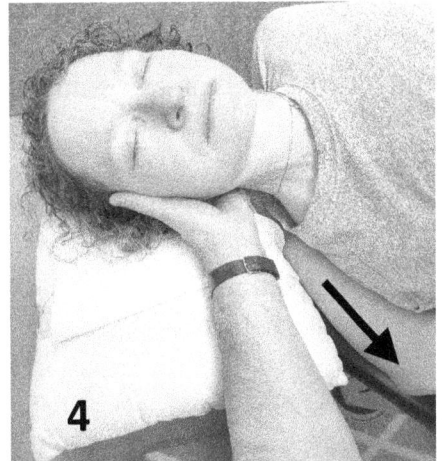

4. Suddenly pull the right contact hand on the first rib, while keeping the head immobile. The tug should be made along the axis of the forearm applying the mobilization.

## Second, Third, and Fourth Ribs

In this example, the restriction is on the right.

Patient position: Prone

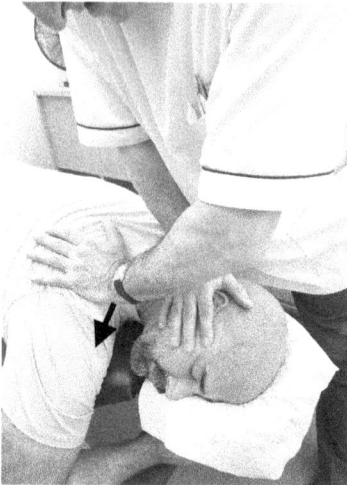

Technic:
1. Stand at the head of the table. Lift the head with both hands, producing extension of the cervicals.
2. Now side bend to the left to a comfortable degree. Communicate with patient about any discomfort. The chin should come to rest on the table if the position is good.
3. Now place your left hand on the temporal bone and rotate the occiput away from the restricted side (in this case, it is right rotation).
4. Continue the right rotation until you see the patient's right shoulder begin to rise.
5. Place your right hand on the ribs and thrust downward toward the table.

# RIBS

## Fifth through Twelfth Ribs

In this example, the restriction is on the left.

Patient position: Lateral recumbent position with the arms folded across the chest

Technic:
1. Sit on the edge of the table facing patient.
2. Pass the left hand under the patient's head and support the upper cervical and occipital region.
3. Make contact with the other hand over the transverse processes of the vertebrae to which the ribs are attached. The ribs themselves will not be the target.
4. Side bend the cervical column toward you and rotate it away from you. Feel for the barrier to further motion.
5. When the optimal tension has been established, make a thrust against the transverse processes toward the midline. This causes a separation of the costotransverse joints, and a gliding movement of the costovertebral joints. The ribs should articulate differently after this indirect mobilization.

# SCOLIOSIS MANEUVERS

The springing-type maneuvers shown here have a cumulative effect in reducing scoliosis.

**Maneuver #1**

Patient position: Lateral recumbent position on the side of convexity, with the legs flexed.

Technic:

1. Stand at the side of the table and further flex patient's lower legs against the thighs, and move the thighs up to the abdomen.
2. Drop the legs over the side of the table and let them hang.
3. Press down on the legs while the other hand grasps the lumbar spine.
4. Make several springing maneuvers in this way to cause rotation that augments the pull on the curve.

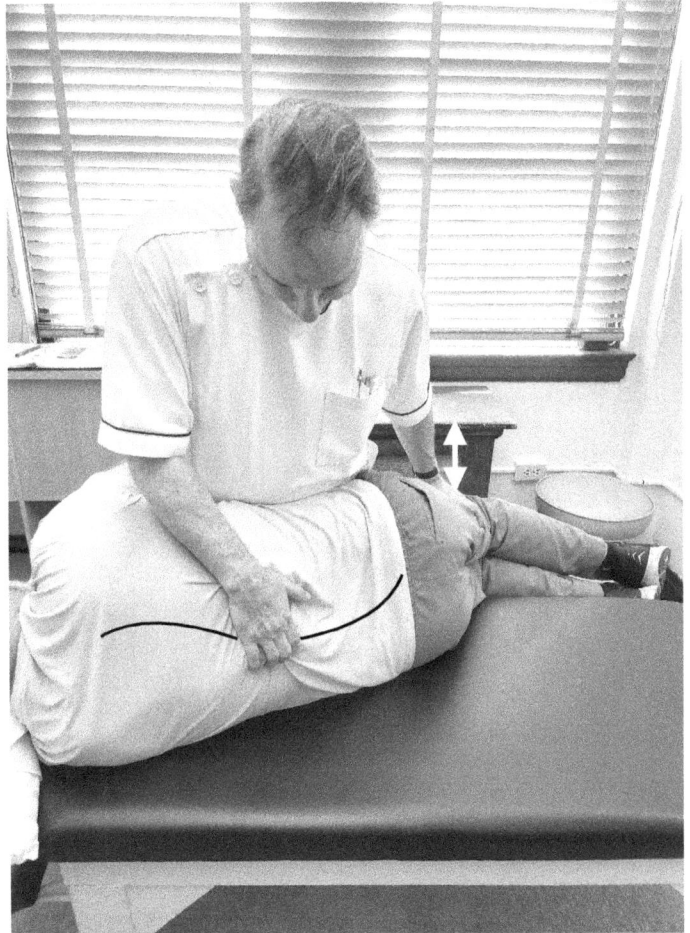

## Maneuver #2

Patient position: Lateral recumbent position on the side of concavity, with the top leg dropped off the table.

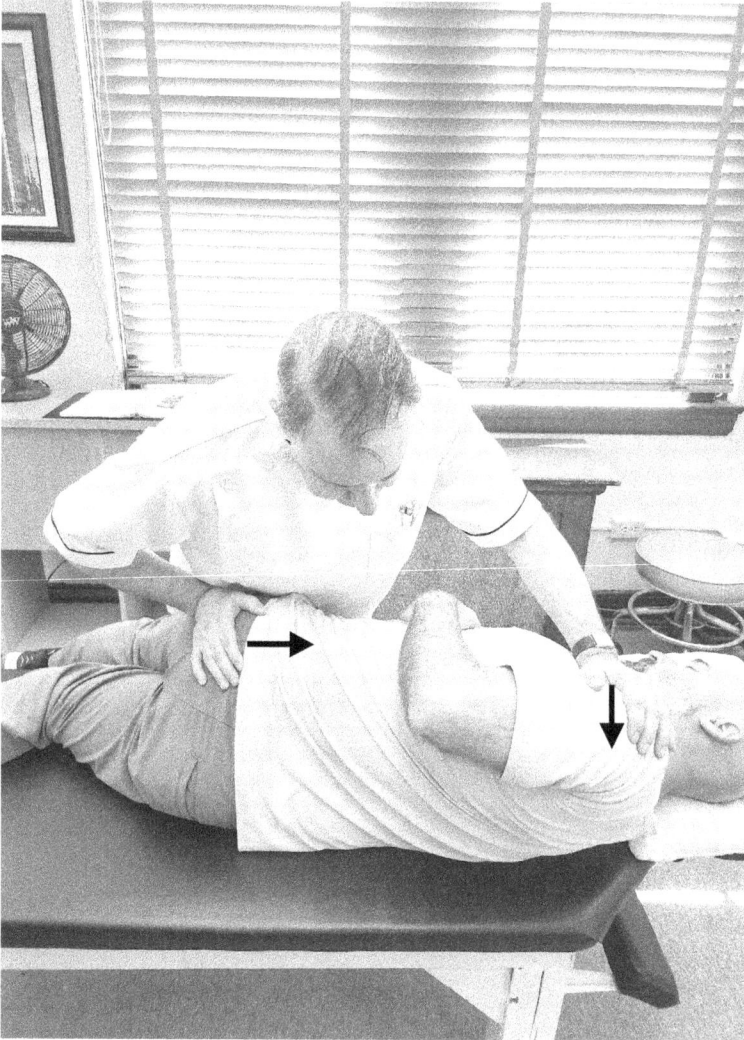

Technic:
1. Stand at the side of the table facing patient. Secure one hand to the patient's anterior shoulder.
2. Place the other hand against the ischial tuberosity.
3. While pushing the shoulder in a posterior direction, press down on the legs with the other hand.
4. Make a thrusting move on the ischial tuberosity in a cephalic direction.

# LUMBAR MANEUVERS

## ASSESSMENT

### LUMBO-SACRAL SPINE EXAM

1. **Check the lumbar curve for normal, reduced, or excessive lordosis.**

    **a.** Normal lumbar lordosis
    **b.** Decreased lumbar curve (left illustration)
    **c.** Increased lumbar lordosis (right illustration)

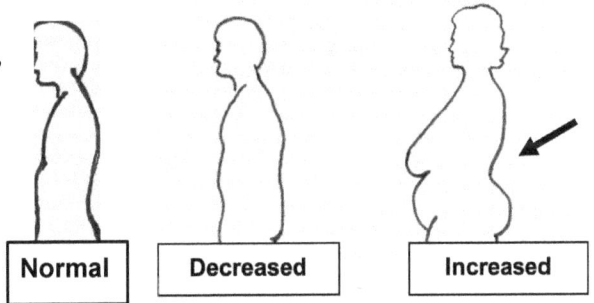

Normal    Decreased    Increased

2. **Check for decreased lumbar range of motion.**

    **a.** Ask the patient to bend forward and try to touch the floor with his fingers. Make note of the angle of the bend and the distance from the fingers to the floor if they do not touch.
    **b.** Have the patient bend backward as far as he can, and steady him with your hand to prevent a fall. Measure the degree of back bending and record it. Normal extension is 30 degrees.

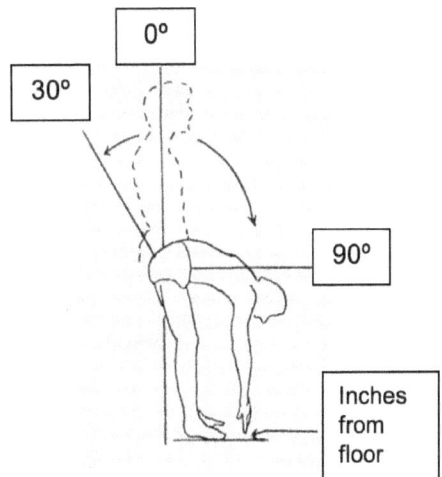

0°

30°

90°

Inches from floor

61

**3. Check for tenderness:** Touch the spinous processes and make a note of any that are tender to palpation. Palpate the paraspinal muscles as well and record if there is any tenderness, rigidity, or obvious spasm in the musculature, and where.

**4. Check for CVA tenderness:**
Place one palm on patient's back over the costovertebral angle (CVA) and strike back of hand with the other fist (**Murphy's renal test**). Sharp pain indicates kidney inflammation. Check both sides. Many cases of low back pain are actually referred from the kidneys

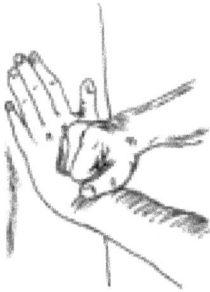

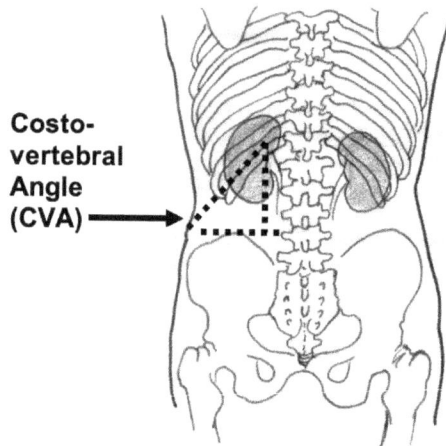

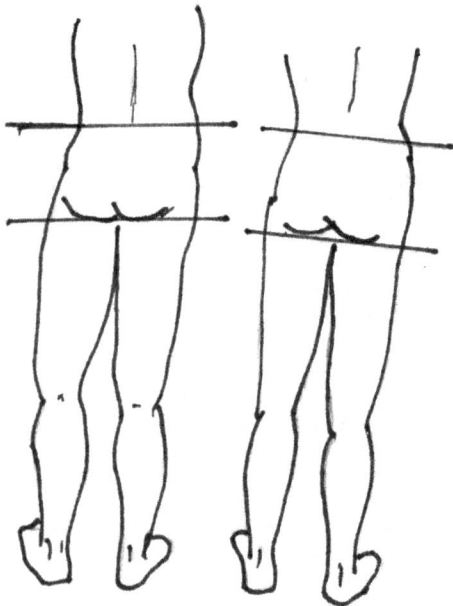

Costo-
vertebral
Angle
(CVA) —→

**5. Check for level iliac crests and buttocks:**
Observe patient from the rear and make note of whether or not one iliac crest is higher, or gluteal crease is higher. Make a note of any abnormal finding.

**6. In cases of low back pain, perform the following tests:**

**Tripod Test**
Grasp patient's ankle and hold down the thigh with the other hand. Quickly extend the leg without warning, as in illustration. If hamstrings are restricted, the patient will immediately resist and the torso will jerk posteriorly to avoid the stretch. If Tripod test is positive, perform Straight Leg Test (SLR or Lasegue Test) to confirm nerve compression or discopathy. If Tripod Test is negative in a patient with exaggerated claims of pain and disability, patient may be a malingerer.

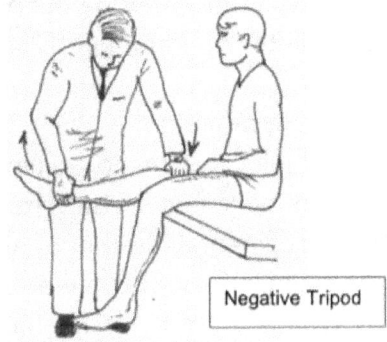

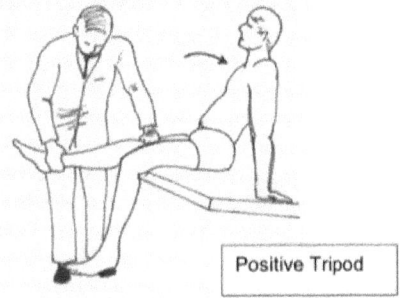

Negative Tripod

Positive Tripod

**Straight Leg Raise** (Lasegue'sTest )
With patient supine, leg is held in extension and slowly raised, with foot dorsiflexed. Radiating pain in the distribution of the nerve root (to below the knee) suggests sciatica (**Lasegue's sign**).

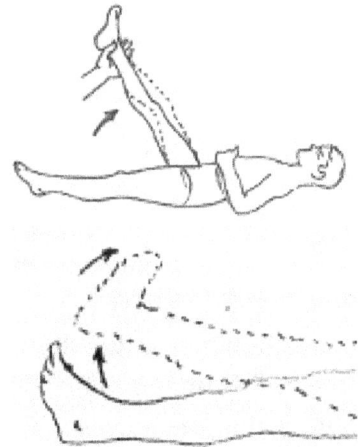

With patient supine, leg is held in extension and slowly raised, with foot dorsiflexed. Pain that prevents lifting to 10 degrees is a positive **Demianoff's sign** and occurs in low back syndromes and contracted hamstrings.

**Thomas' test.** Flexion contractures of the hip can be obscured by excessive lumbar lordosis. Have patent lie supine, fully extending one leg flat on the exam table and flex the other leg, drawing the knee to the chest. Operator can assist. Observe the patient's ability to keep the extended leg flat on the table or dangling over the edge. If the leg involuntarily flexes, it indicates Psoas muscle contracture. Treatment of the same can be accomplished by applying resistance to the extended leg

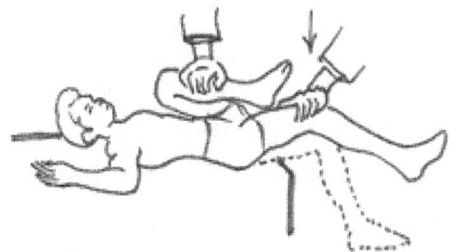

as in the illustration, asking the patient to intermittently flex against the resistance, then relax while the operator gently stretches the psoas.

## Sacroiliac dysfunction

Sacroiliac joint dysfunction typically causes the patient to make deliberate movements, rising from a sitting position in one unit, without segmental flexion of the spine.    Patient will try to support himself with his hands on the surface from which he is rising (Amoss's Sign).    The hand will usually be instinctively placed on the affected area in an attempt to immobilize it.

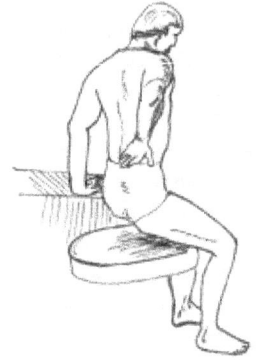

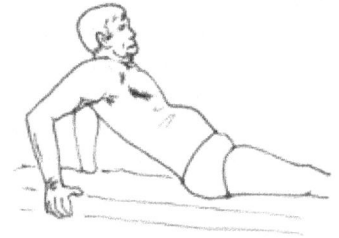

**Patrick's test** (also known as the FABERE test: Flexion, Abduction, External Rotation and Extension).  Ask the patient to relax and not try to move leg.   Move patient's leg passively through this maneuver and note any pain and guarding. Press gently against the knee while anchoring the opposite hip as in the illustration. Hip pain that is referred from another location will not appear during this maneuver.   Pain that is elicited is a positive FABERE or Patrick's test.   Sacroiliitis is suggested by this finding.

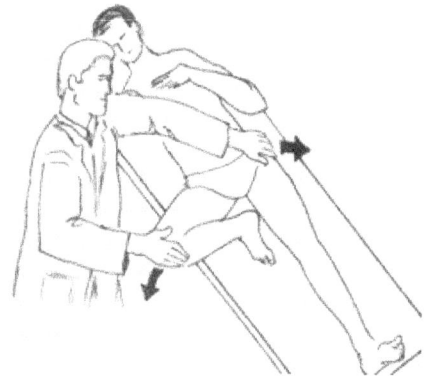

**Piriformis test**   With patient lying prone, flex the leg on the affected side to 90º, and draw the lower leg toward you, gripping just superior to the ankle joint. At the same time, stabilize the sacrum with the other hand so that the pelvis does not rotate with the action.   Undue stiffness and pain from this torque action indicates Piriformis muscle contraction and is present in sciatica and low back syndromes.   The Piriformis can be stretched with this maneuver as a therapeutic measure as well.

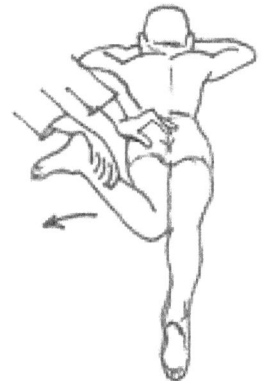

**Erichsen's test**  With patient standing facing you, grasp the iliac bones and press them towards each other.  Pain is a positive sign of sacroiliac disease or early spondylolitic arthritis.

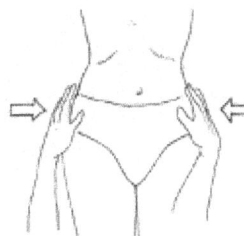

**Trendelenburg hip test**  Patient stands on the side to be tested and raises the other leg off the floor.  Examiner observes from behind.  Observation of the gluteal creases will ordinarily show the crease of the raised leg rise.  If it remains level or drops, it is indicative of gluteus medius weakness on the affected side (or congenital hip dislocation), and is a positive Trendelenburg sign.

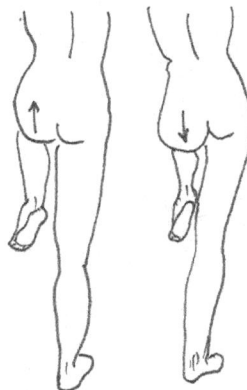

| Normal | Positive Trendelenburg |

**Guide To Lumbar Nerve Root Compression / Herniated Nucleus Pulposus**

| Nerve Root | L1 | L2 | L3 | L4 | L5 | S1 |
|---|---|---|---|---|---|---|
| Pain | | | | | | |
| Numbness | X | X | X | | | |
| Motor Weakness | X | Slight weakness on extension of quadriceps | Pronounced weakness on extension of quadriceps | Quadriceps extension | Dorsiflexion of Great Toe and Foot | Plantar Flexion of Great Toe and Foot |
| Exam | X | Squat & Rise | Squat & Rise | Squat & Rise | Heel Walking | Toe Walking |
| Reflex | X | Normal or ↓ Suprapatellar | ↓ Suprapatellar or patellar | ↓ Knee Jerk | No Test Reliable. | ↓ Ankle Jerk |

65

## Lumbosacral Soft Tissue Technic

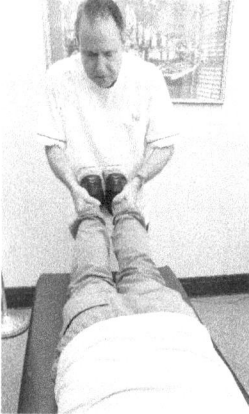

This is a procedure recommended in any new case of low back pain.

Patient is prone. Check the length of both legs. A discrepancy in leg length in the majority of cases is the result of sacroiliac (SI Joint) misalignment and restriction.

Stand on the contralateral side from the short leg. Place one hand firmly on the opposite posterior superior iliac spine (PSIS). The other hand makes contact at the knee of the short leg, and lifts the leg, revolving it in a circular motion. Make wide circles five or six times, then move the hip contact hand superiorly to press at the L4-L5 level. Make the circular movements again, and then move the contact hand up to the L3-L4 level and repeat. Move superiorly again to the L2-L3 level and repeat. Then reverse direction and repeat the entire process in reverse order until you return to the ASIS.

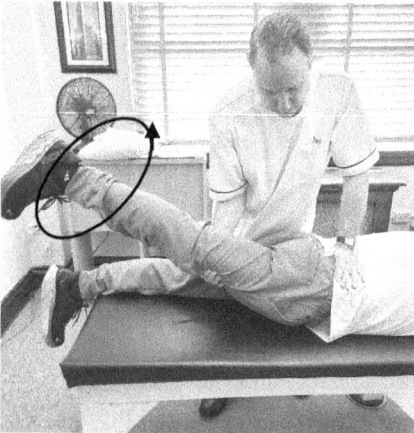

Check leg length again. If corrected, no further treatment is needed. If not corrected, the joint may need to be given mobilization with impulse (See section on **sacral / hip maneuvers**).

It sometimes happens that the above maneuver results in an over-correction of sorts, and the formerly short leg is now long. In such an event, repeat the procedure on the opposite side, with fewer circular motions, and then check leg length. Note: There are anatomical short legs, caused by injury, complications of delivery at birth, or diseases like polio. But the vast majority of short leg manifestations are functional, not anatomical.

## Rotation Correction

For a right lumbar rotation, position the patient in a lateral recumbent posture with knees flexed (Sim's position), on the patient's right side. Stand in front of patient and secure a grip just superior to the bottom knee. Place the other hand on the (close) left scapula. Then lift the thighs off the table while maintaining pressure on the scapula. Lower the thighs, then lift again, rhythmically, several times. Re-assess the hips afterward to see if the rotation is resolved. For a left lumbar rotation, reverse the instructions.

## Spinal Stretch

A preparatory maneuver prior to mobilization with impulse.

Using one hand to drag the tissues caudally and the other in a cephalic direction, the soft tissue of the spine is stretched in segments. Hold each stretch for 7 seconds or so, then move the hands to new positions and repeat until the full spine is stretched. The longissimus, the spinalis, and the iliocostalis muscles are affected by this, as well as the fascia.

Depending on preference, you can use a wide "open" positioning or a crossed positioning.

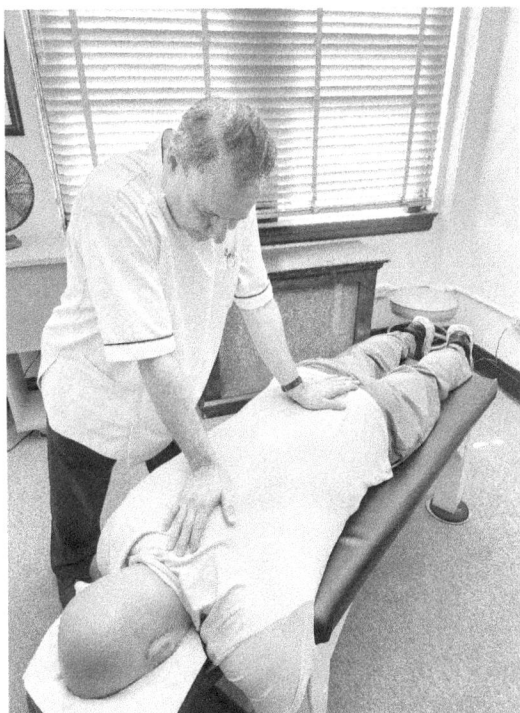

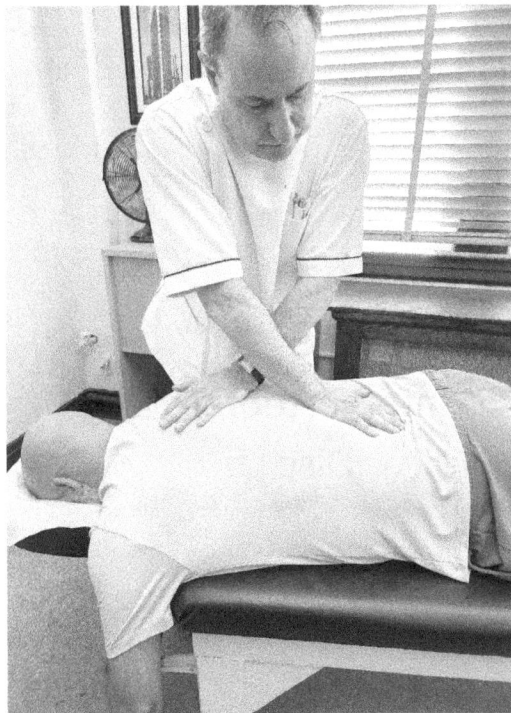

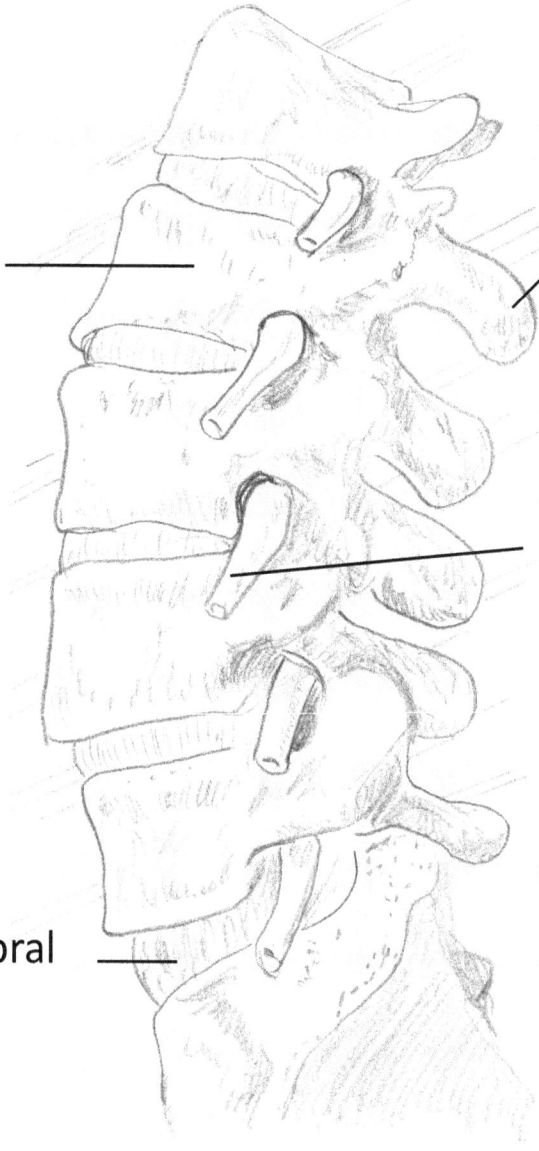

Vertebra Body

Spinous Process

Nerve Root

Intervertebral Disc

# LUMBAR #1   **Prone Upper Lumbar Thrust**

Site of restriction:  L1-L3

Patient position:  Prone

Technic:
1. Stand on the side opposite the restriction.
2. Slide one hand under the patient's axilla so that you elevate the shoulder from the table.
3. With the other hand, contact the transverse process of the lower of the vertebrae involved in the restriction. This is on the same side as the elevated shoulder. Contact is made with the hypothenar eminence and the fingers point in a cephalic direction.
4. While drawing up on patient's shoulder, thrust down toward the table and slightly laterally.

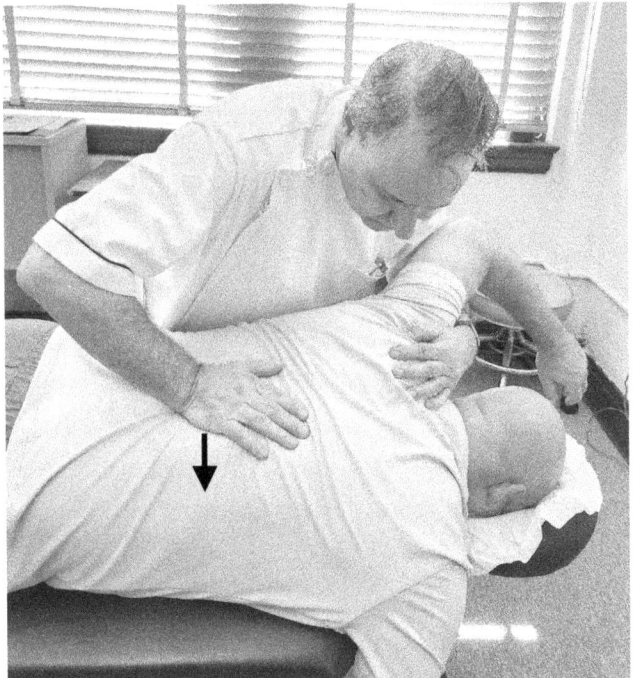

# LUMBAR #2    Prone Upper Lumbar Thrust, variation

This maneuver is better for smaller doctors than the previous one due to improved leverage.

Site of restriction: L1-L3

Patient position: Prone

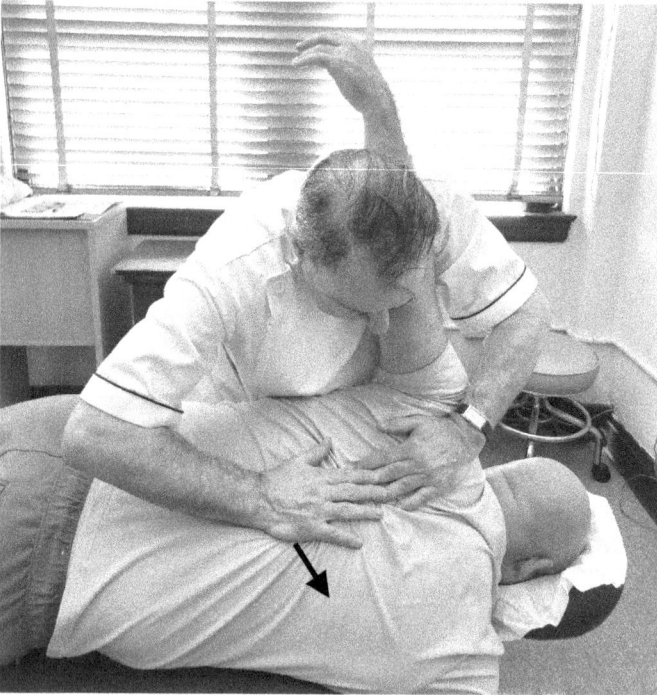

Technic:

1. Position is the same as Lumbar #1, except that the arm is passed under patient's shoulder and your hands are clasped together. There is more leverage in elevating the shoulder in this way.

2. The cephalic hand aims at the target vertebra transverse process with the hypothenar eminence, just off the fingertips of the lower hand.

3. The caudal hand delivers a thrust directed down and slightly cephalic.

# LUMBAR #3   **Prone Upper Lumbar Thrust with Rotation**

Site of restriction:  L1-L3

Patient position:  Prone

Technic:
1. Stand on the side opposite the restriction.
2. Flex the patient's leg on the side of the restriction to 90 degrees and draw it over the other leg, holding against the proximal popliteal space.   By applying pressure on the ankle, rotation from below is produced.
3. With the other hand, contact the transverse process of the upper vertebra in the restriction.  Contact is made with the thenar eminence. Fingers are perpen-dicular to the spine.  Do not flex the fingers.
4. Deliver a thrust down toward the table and somewhat laterally.

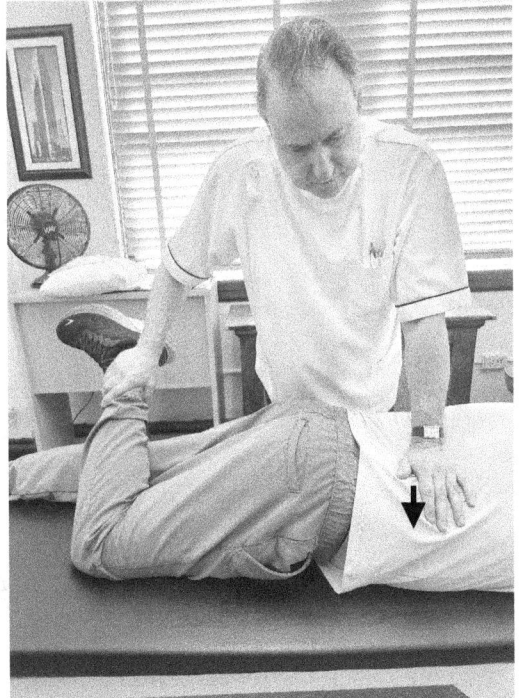

# LUMBAR #4    Supine Lumbar Lift

Site of restriction:  L3-L5

Patient position:  Supine

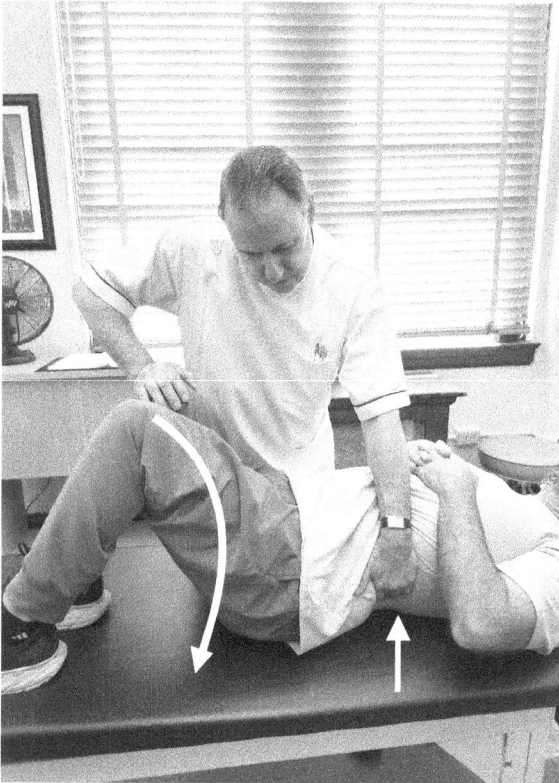

Technic:
1. Patient lies supine with the legs drawn up and feet on the table.
2. Stand on the side opposite the restriction.  Grasp the knees with your close hand and pull them toward you.
3. Using this increased rotation, reach with the other hand and grasp the patient's contralateral posterior superior iliac spine (PSIS).
4. Keep the hip elevated while you push the legs toward the affected side.

# LUMBAR #5    **Prone Lumbar Lift**

Site of restriction:  L3-L5

Patient position:  Prone

Technic:
1. Stand at the side of the table.
2. Place one hand on the lower lumbar transverse processes and give a deep pressure downward through the hypothenar eminence.
3. Grasp the contralateral anterior superior iliac spine (ASIS).  Since this is generally a ticklish area, it helps to use a couple folds of toweling to cushion this grip.
4. Pull upwards on the ASIS while maintaining the downward pressure on the transverse processes.
5. When the barrier is reached, apply impulse P-A to the lumbar contact to make the mobilization.

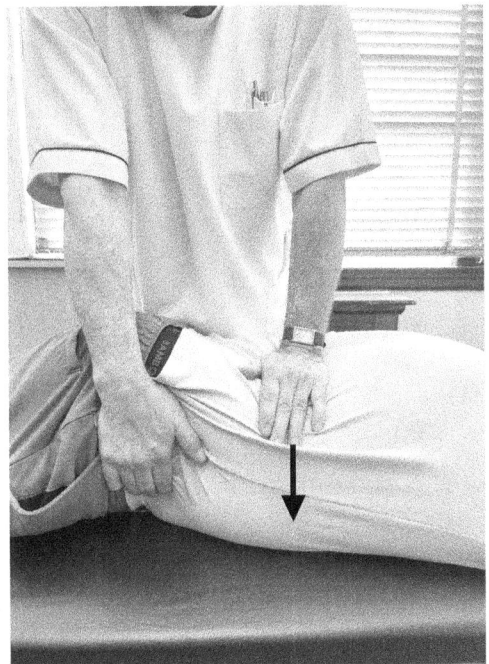

# LUMBAR #6    "Kick Start" Lumbar Roll

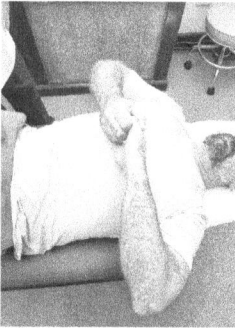

Site of restriction:  L2-L5

Patient position:  Lateral recumbent

Technic:

1.Stand at the side of the table facing the patient, who is in a right lateral recumbent posture.

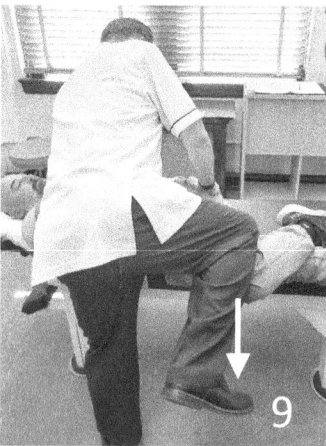

2.Flex patient's top leg and position the ankle behind the other popliteal space.   The other leg should be relatively straight.

3.Ask patient to lock fingers together as illustrated in top photo.

4.Pull on the bottom arm in order to place the torso in a more supine presentation and increase the rotation.

5.Make certain patient's face is turned to neutral (facing same direction as the chest).

6.Ask patient to inhale.

7.Grasp the far elbow of the patient with your left hand and make a lateral pressure to fix the torso in neutral.

8.Place your right hand on the posterior superior iliac spine (PSIS).

9.Place your right knee in the popliteal space of the top leg, while raising up the heel of your left foot off the floor.

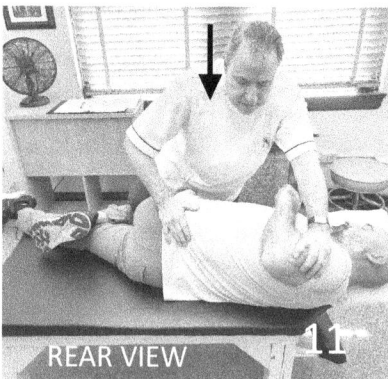

REAR VIEW

10. As patient exhales, lower your right knee (and therefore the patient's leg) until you encounter the barrier.

11. When you have engaged the barrier, give a kick toward the floor (just as you would kick start a motorcycle) and simultaneously drop the left heel back onto the floor, as you maintain pressure on the PSIS and the patient's arms.

This maneuver uses very powerful muscles to create the mobilization, and is thus ideal for the smaller practitioner.

# LUMBAR #7 Hooking Lumbar Roll

Site of restriction: L2-L5 as well as SI joint

Patient position: Lateral recumbent

Technic:
1. Stand at side of table facing patient who is in a lateral posture similar to Lumbar #6, except that the top leg is allowed to hand down off the table.
2. Ask patient to lock fingers together as illustrated.
3. Pull on the bottom arm in order to adjust the torso in a more supine presentation if needed.
4. Push the far elbow to create rotation in the opposite direction from the lumbar spine and place your other hand on the PSIS.
5. Have patient breathe in and out.
6. During the exhale, hook your leg in the popliteal space of the dangling leg and suddenly pull it in the direction of the head of the table.
7. Simultaneously with the leg movement, thrust down on the PSIS and push the patient's arms a but farther to the side, increasing the rotation. His upper body will be rotated away from you, and his lower body toward you.

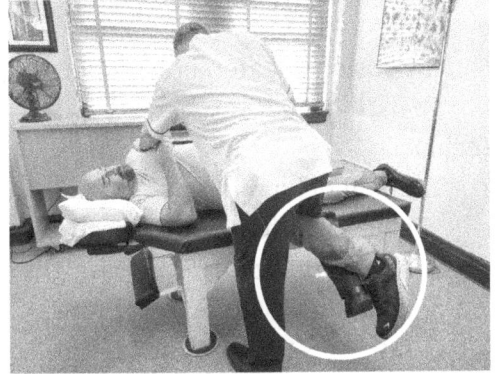

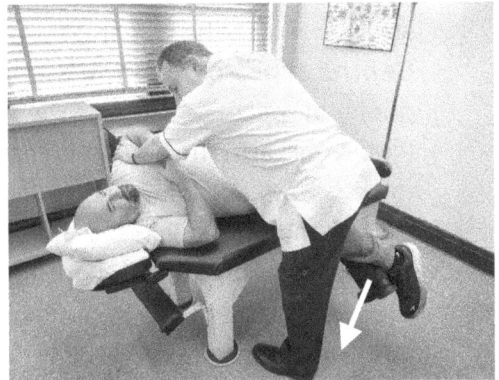

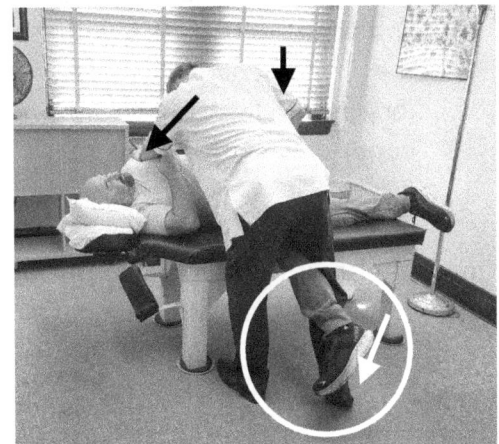

# LUMBAR #8    Reverse Lumbar Roll

Site of restriction:  L2-L5 as well as SI joint

Patient position:  Lateral recumbent

Technic:
1. Stand behind the patient and have him fold his arms across his chest, gripping his elbows.  A folded towel can be placed on the chest to minimize pressure.
2. Assure that the body is straight on the table with no rotation.
3. Have the patient bend the top leg 90 degrees at the hip and keep the bottom leg straight.  Place the top ankle behind the other leg's popliteal space.
4. Pass your arm through his folded arms and place your other hand on the PSIS.
5. Have patient breathe and on the exhale, rotate the lower body and apply impulse by pulling his arms toward you and thrusting the PSIS with the hypothenar eminence (or specifically, the pisiform bone) down the axis of the femur.

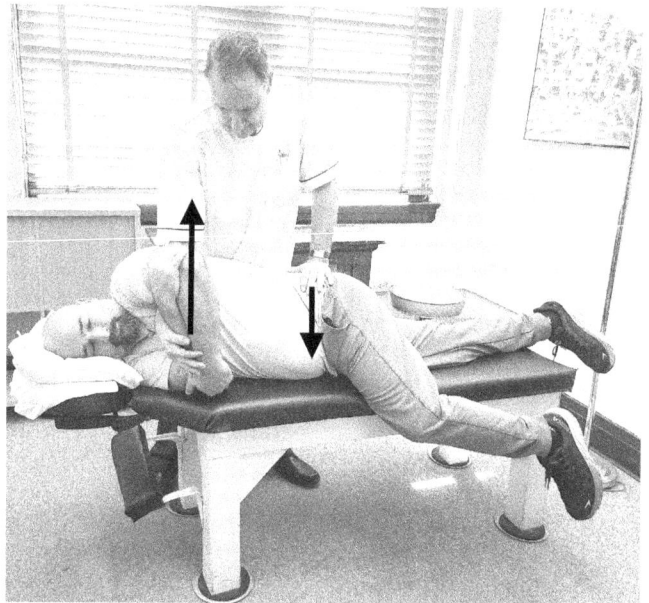

One can also, if needed, apply this maneuver with the leg dangling over the table as seen.  This is the same as in Lumbar #7.

# LUMBAR #9    **Standard Lumbar Rotation Maneuver**

Site of restriction:  L2-L5 as well as SI joint

Patient position:  Supine

Technic:

1. Stand to the side of the patient and have him fold his arms across his chest, gripping his elbows.
2. Flex the far leg 90 degrees at the hip and place it in adduction.  Place the top ankle behind the other leg's popliteal space.
3. Pass your cephalic arm through his folded arms and place it on the area to be treated.  Place your other hand on the PSIS.

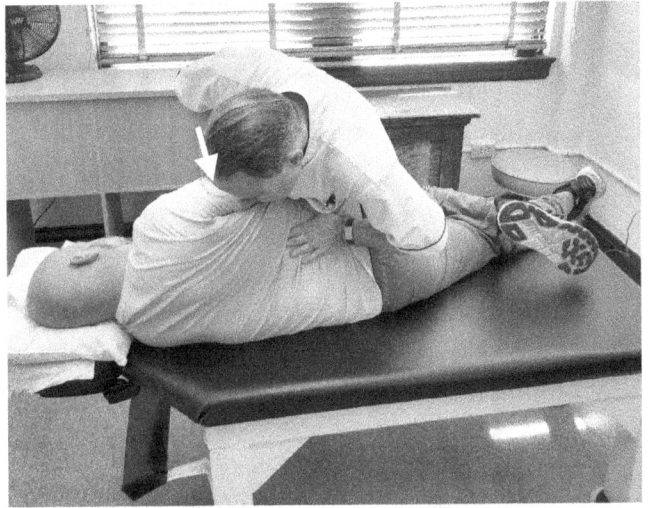

4. Have patient breathe, and on the exhale, rotate the lower body and find the barrier.  At the end of the exhalation, move him into further rotation by applying impulse by pulling his ilium toward you and making an A-P impulse against his anterior shoulder with your elbow.  Your body should rotate as the caudal elbow moves posteriorly.  Your body must be leaning as far over the patient's body as possible, so that your sternum is on a line above the lumbar spine.

# LUMBAR #10   Standard Lumbar Rotation Maneuver, variation

Site of restriction:  L2-L5 as well as SI joint

Patient position:  Supine

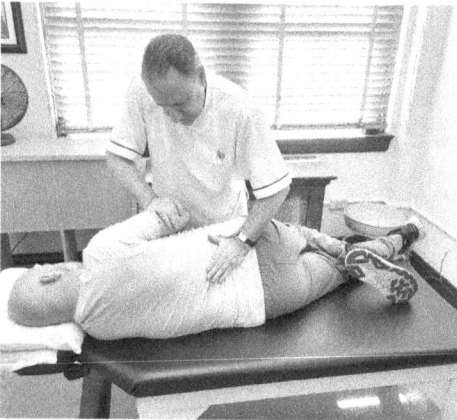

Technic:

1. As for Lumbar #9, stand to the side of the patient and have him fold his arms across his chest, gripping his elbows.

2. Flex the far leg 90 degrees at the hip and place it in adduction.  Place the top ankle behind the other leg's popliteal space.

3. Pass your cephalic arm through his folded arms and place it on the area to be treated. Place your other hand on top of the hand.  Your elbow should be firmly against the PSIS.

4. Have patient breathe, and on the exhale, roll the patient's body toward you as though to roll him off the edge of the table.  Find the barrier. At the end of the exhalation, drop your weight and apply impulse to the PSIS with your elbow along the axis of the femur.  As you do this, your top hand will disengage.  Your body should be leaning over as in Lumbar #9, and rotated a bit as the caudal elbow make its P-A thrust.

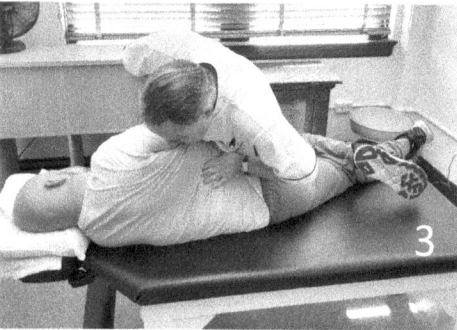

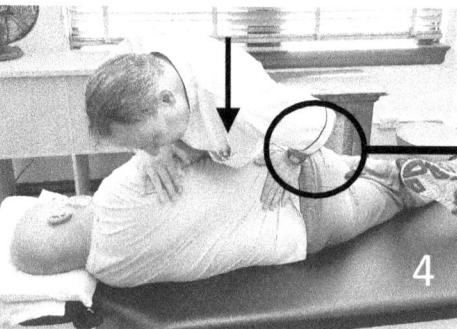

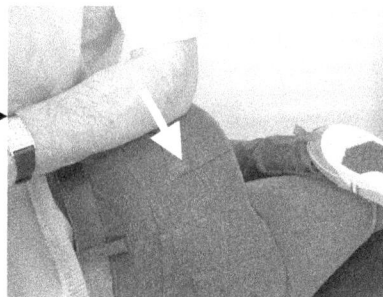

# LUMBAR #11   **Prone Lumbar Flexion Release**

Site of restriction:  L1-L5, in a flexion restriction

Patient position:  Prone with patient resting on elbows, arms crossed

When there is pain in the lumbar region on forward bending, determine the tender vertebra and aim your maneuver at this target.

Technic:
1. The patient's ankles should hang free of the table.  Tell patient to place the neck in a relaxed position.
2. Grasp the ipsilateral calf with one hand, and with the other hand make a contact on the lower of the two vertebrae in restriction.
3. Instruct the patient to raise the head slowly.  As he begins, thrust down with the contact hand in a cephalic direction.

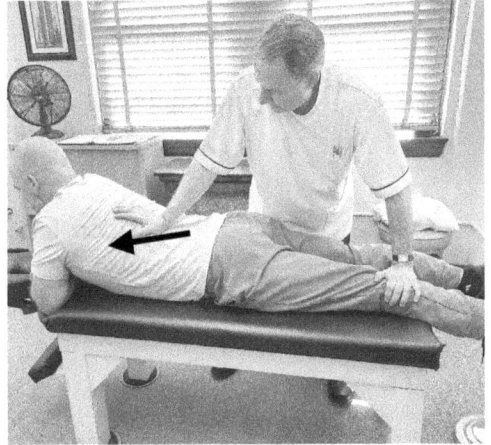

# DISC PROLAPSE / HERNIATION

### Disc prolapse / herniation

While the orthopedist relies on MRI for confirmation, the naturopath can fairly reliably assess this condition.

1. Unequal leg length
2. Rotation of L5 (likely on the side of a posterior ilium)
3. Unequal level of pubic symphysis (high side = side of posterior ilium)
4. Palpatory assessment of disc space (a thin disc does *not* necessarily imply herniation)
5. Positive Tripod Test, Lasegue Test (described in **Assessment**)

### Troedssen Maneuver

Site of restriction:  L3-L5 discopathy

Patient position:  Supine, ideally with cervical traction applied

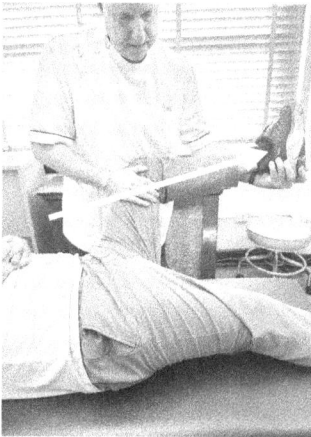

Technic:
1.Stand at the foot of the table and flex the patient's knee on the abdomen.
2.Tell patient to kick outward from there (extend the leg).
3.Relax the flexion you have created as he kicks, and accentuate the kick with your hands.  Grasp the knee with one hand and the ankle with the other.
4.Perform the augmented kick 10 times, then repeat with the other leg.

The action of this maneuver is the forceful stretching of the disc and a pumping of fluid into the spinal segments.

While this book is focused on maneuvers that do not require any special equipment, a word should be made of the Cox Flexion/Distraction technic.  This development from Chiropractic is practically unrivaled for decompression of prolapsed or herniated discs. It requires a special table, which can be quite expensive, but the technic is very simple and reliable, and not unpleasant for the patient.

# SECTION SIX

## SACRAL / HIP ( INNOMINATE ) MANEUVERS

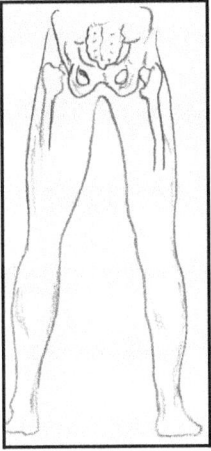

Most joint pain in this region that you will encounter will not stem from specific changes in the trochanter or acetabulum, i.e., the "ball and socket" hip joint. Rather, changes in the positioning of the ilium and ischium, on one or both sides, will present as "hip" pain.

Sacroiliac (SI) joint dysfunction is characterized by pain and stiffness in the region connecting the sacrum and ilii (hip bones). This condition can cause low back pain, buttock pain, and often radicular leg pain, radiating down the posterior thigh.

From an examination of the bony structures, one can see how the sciatic nerve can be impinged.

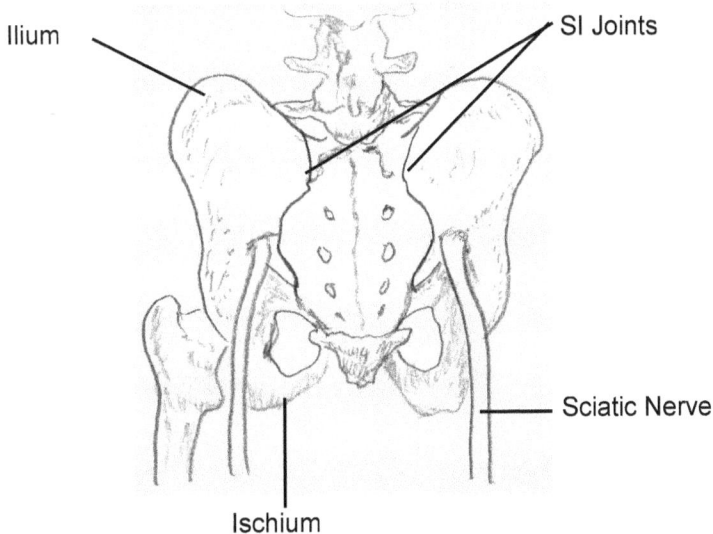

Ilium

SI Joints

Sciatic Nerve

Ischium

There are many contributing factors for SI Joint dysfunction, but one must first eliminate ligamentous laxity as a cause. A good history and examination should reveal any hypermobility of the joints. With laxity of the ligaments, mobilization with impulse may be contraindicated.

The ligaments you are dealing with can be visualized here.

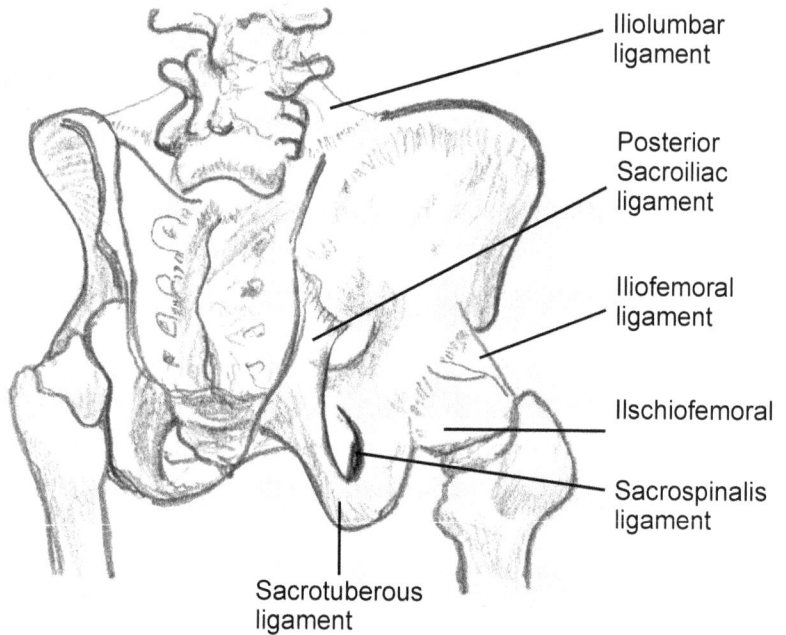

Iliolumbar ligament

Posterior Sacroiliac ligament

Iliofemoral ligament

Ilschiofemoral

Sacrospinalis ligament

Sacrotuberous ligament

Muscular imbalances, in the Piriformis and / or Gluteal muscles are the most frequent cause. Tension in the lumbar region can contribute to, or result from, SI Joint pain. Sometimes trauma is the precipitating factor, such as a fall landing on the buttocks. Also chronic autoimmune disease can cause this dysfunction. And sometimes there will be a true "hip joint" dysfunction, i.e., femoral-acetabluar impingement.

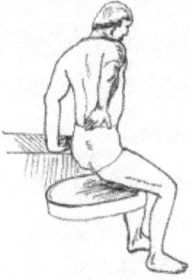

Diagnostically, the patient's gait and seated posture will inform you even before you palpate the illii. As discussed in Section 5, sacroiliac joint dysfunction typically causes the patient to make deliberate movements, rising from a sitting position in one unit, without segmental flexion of the spine. Patient will try to support himself with his hands on the surface from which he is rising (Amoss's Sign). The hand will usually be instinctively placed on the affected area in an attempt to immobilize it. The patient will typically report pain at, or inferomedial to, the PSIS

## Typical clinical presentation

- Unequal iliac crest height
- Unequal weight-bearing when standing
- Painful "catching" or increased pain ipsilaterally during stance phase
- Decreased hip extension (resulting in shortened contralateral stride length)
- Gluteus medius weakness
- Tight iliopsoas, piriformis, and hamstrings

There are various tests for sacroiliac joint disorders but no agreed-upon single standard. Many tests are actually poor at revealing joint restriction at that site. However, the so-called "Stork Test" has been historically relied upon. It is simple and not time consuming.

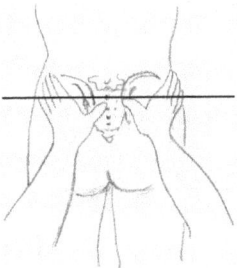

Abnormal stork test

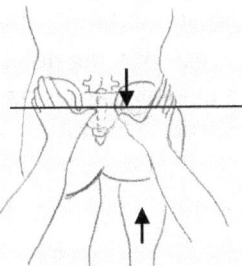

Normal stork test

### Stork Test (or Gillet Test)

Have the patient standing with a hand on the table or other furniture for stabilization. Locate the SI Joint on the left side. Place the pad of your right thumb against the right PSIS and the left thumb around one inch medial, over S2. The tips of the thumbs face each other on a horizontal plane. Have the patient life the right knee as high as they can (at least 90º). It should be as high as possible to initiate motion in the joint. A normal test will show the PSIS dropping a bit inferiorly and slightly medially. When it does not, the joint is not moving and there is restriction. Restriction keeps the sacrum and the PSIS level during the motion. Repeat test on the other side if the patient's pain is not localized.

Now put your attention on the sacral side of the joint. Make the same two-thumb contact as before and have the patient raise the contralateral knee. See if the sacral side, under your right thumb, moves inferiorly. This is a normal finding. If it does not move, once again the joint is "stuck". Perform on the patient's other side and record your findings.

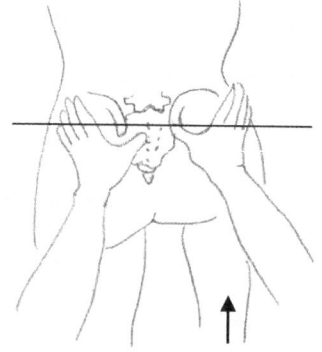

Positive stork test: Thumb does not move inferiorly, but possibly superiorly

Not all pain is necessarily due to restriction. Note that there may be cases of hypermobility in the joints that create instability and the sacroiliac joint is no exception. Such conditions are not amenable to impulse-style mobilizations and require a more comprehensive treatment. However, a hypermobile joint will also cause a positive finding on the Stork Test. For this and other reasons, the test does not have a high degree of reliability and is discouraged in some physiotherapy circles. But because naturopaths have many tools in their repertoire, an overall assessment can boost the accuracy of any individual test for determining the appropriate treatment.

The ilium can also be restricted or fixed in a superior direction (upslip) or inferior direction (downslip). If the ilium does not move in either direction, it is usually due to an upslip.

As we have seen already in the previous chapter, there are many maneuvers to reduce a malposition of the sacroiliac joint, including some involving the lumbar spine. Sacroiliac joint dysfunction is a restriction that presents very often in clinical practice. Many times lumbar maneuvers are not effective for lumbar pain because the SI joint still needs to be freed. However, rotation of L5 often accompanies SI joint dysfunction. This places the PSIS in a posterior position. When the ilium slips backwards, it pulls on the ileolumbar ligaments, inducing rotation of the body of L5 and / or L4 on the side of the slip.

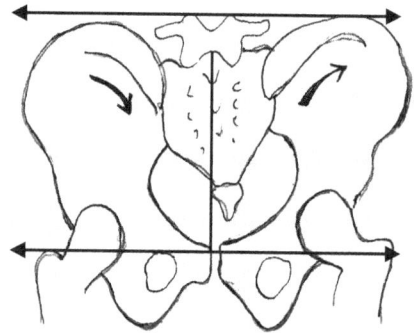

Left posterior ilium. Frontal view of pelvic torsion visualized through the axis of the iliac crests and the pubic synthesis. Note uneven iliac crests and trochanters, and sacral tilt.

Checking leg length is the first thing to be done. SI joint dysfunction typically produces a short leg presentation on the painful side. Posterior-inferior (P-I) malposition is the usual presentation. However, it has been argued that leg length measurement should not be the criterion for assessing SI joint malposition and it goes without saying that palpation is always the best means of establishing the direction a corrective move should take.

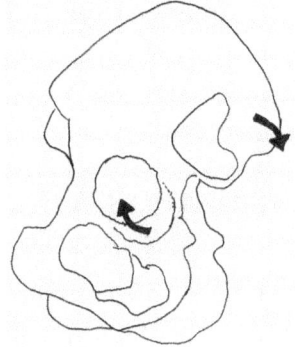

In the side view illustration at right, the left ilium has shifted posteriorly to the degree that not only functional short leg results, but there is strain in the pubic symphysis. Pain in the pudenda can be a symptom of SI Joint dysfunction.

If the ilium has shifted anteriorly, the mechanics are the reverse of the illustration. Anterior malposition is said to occur 80% of the time on the right side, for some reason.

In the case of upslip or downslip, palpation of the sacrotuberous ligament can be used to assess. As one can see, the sacrotuberous ligament originates from the sacrum and inserts into the ischial tuberosity. When the ilium is in an upslip position, the ligament will be soft and elastic. When there is a downslip, the ligament is pulled more taut, and often feels almost like bone to the touch. Obviously, a working knowledge of regional anatomy and the development of palpatory skills are essential for accurately evaluating sacroiliac dysfunction. See illustration at right for location.

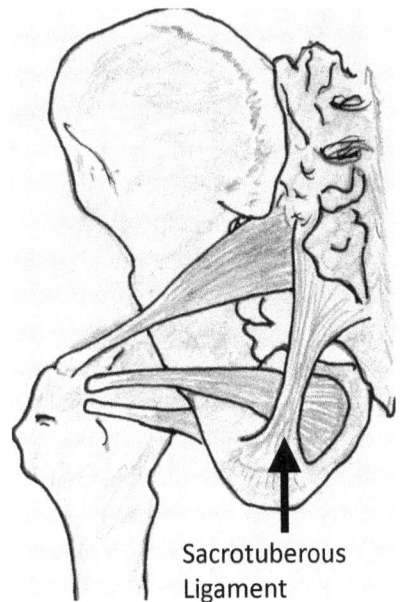

Sacrotuberous Ligament

Returning to the matter of leg length: You may encounter a "double sacroiliac slip", in which case leg length is equal. If leg length is equal and the patient still experiences pain in the hips, it is likely a bilateral restriction, typically an anterior-superior (A-S) restriction or fixation.

While bilateral restrictions are common, they are almost always due to muscular adaptation in the face of thoracic and lumbar spine restrictions. Therefore, assessment and treatment of the thoracolumbar region should precede the sacroiliac treatment. This may not involve mobilization, but can be effected by induced muscular relaxation, by low volt sine wave treatment, or mechanical vibration, or simply soft tissue manual therapies.

## MOBILIZATION WITHOUT IMPULSE

As discussed above, manual therapy or electrotherapy may be applied to the areas with the most muscle tension in the thoracolumbar region.

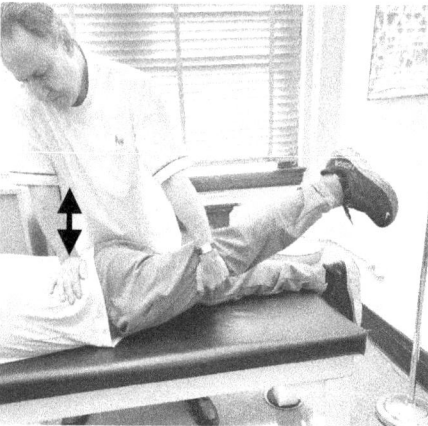

A gentle maneuver without impulse may be applied as follows:

**Prone Scissors Maneuver**

Have patient lie prone. Stand on opposite side from affected side. Raise the leg on the affected side with one hand while pressing on the PSIS with the other. Draw the leg across to the popliteal space of the opposite leg. Maintain the position of the legs while making several "springing" or rocking motions against the PSIS, down and up.

## MOBILIZATION WITH IMPULSE

The basic rule for SI joint treatment is this:

- Assess and determine if the problem is a posterior malposition of the ilium (or ilii, in the case of a bilateral problem), or an anterior malposition, or an upslip or downslip of the innominate.
- Assess and treat any restrictions or myospasm in the thoracolumbar spine before mobilizing the SI joint.
- Posterior position: thrust high on the PSIS
- Anterior position: thrust on the spine of the ischium.
- In both cases, immobilize the sacrum with the other hand during the procedure.

In all sacroiliac cases, take care to first:

1. Test for range of motion
2. Check for unequal leg length
3. Rule out any lower thoracic or lumbar restrictions before moving the sacroiliac

## SIJ #1   Posterior Lift Maneuver

Site of restriction:  SI joint, posterior position

Patient position:  Prone

Technic:

1. Same procedure as for the Prone Scissors Maneuver previously detailed.  Stand on the contralateral side from the restriction.
2. Place the caudal hand under patient's thigh above the patella
3. Place the cephalic hand on the PSIS.  Your fingers will rest on the Gluteus medius.
4. Elevate the thigh while checking for any lumbar muscle contraction.  If so, do not attempt to move the SIJ.
5. Slightly adduct the patient's leg as you elevate it, while at the same time make a rhythmic rocking pressure against the PSIS.  Make several rocking motions.
6. If the time is right, thrust down against the PSIS while being careful to not lower the leg with the other hand.

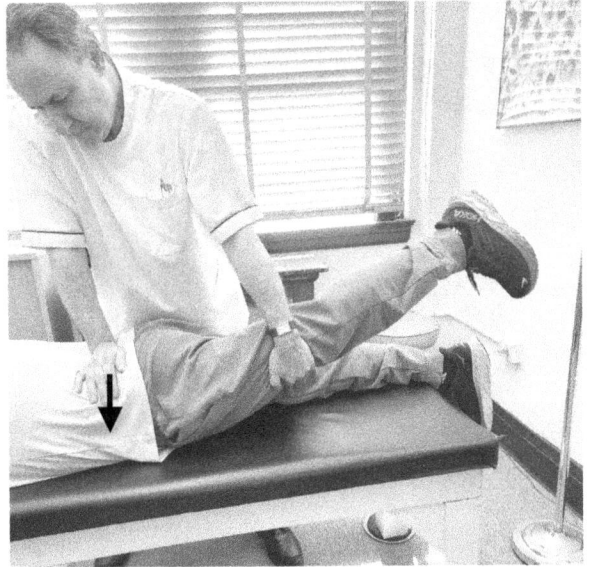

# SIJ #2    Prone Sacroiliac Release

Site of restriction:  SI joint, posterior position, or anterior position*

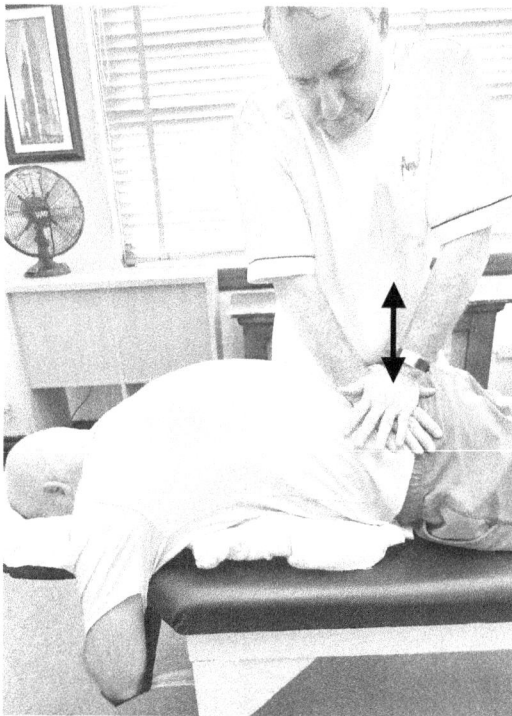

Patient position:   Prone with two pillows under the abdomen and two pillows under the thighs.  The pelvis should be free of the table.

Technic:
1.Stand on the contralateral side.
2.Place one hand just posterior to the PSIS with the other hand reinforcing the contact.
3.Make a few recoiling or "springing" thrusts.

* If the ilium is anterior, perform with the hand placed medial to the PSIS, over the sacrum.

# SIJ #3    Supine Abduction-Extension Release

Site of restriction:  SI joint, posterior position*, or anterior position*

Patient position:  Supine

Technic:
1. Stand on the ipsilateral side.
2. Grasp patient's leg at the ankle with one hand, placing your other hand over the patella.
3. Flex the leg and thigh.
4. Abduct the leg, externally rotating it with both hands.
5. Quickly pull on the ankle and force the leg into extension, thus releasing the sacroiliac.

* If ilium is anterior, adduct the leg instead of abduction and internally rotate it before extension.

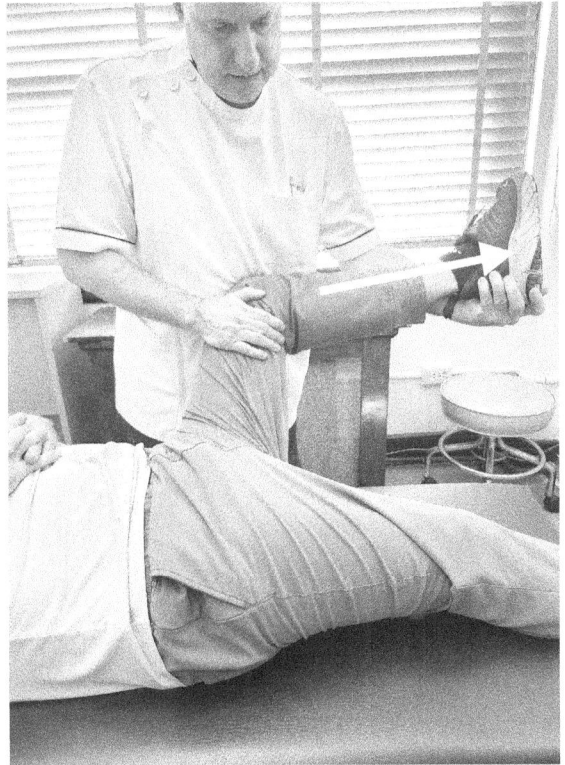

**"Diamond Maneuver"**

# SIJ #4

Site of restriction:  SI joint, posterior or anterior position; pubic joint

Patient position:  Supine

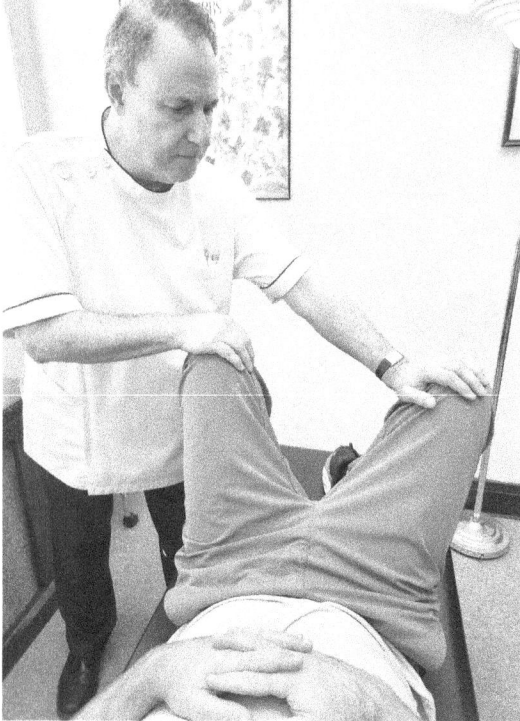

Technic:
1. Have patient flex both thighs and legs.
2. Have patient keep the feet touching each other.
3. Place your hands medially to the knee joints and abduct both knees, causing a diamond-like shape to be created by the gap.
4. Maintain abduction with the hands and ask patient to suddenly extend both legs by kicking his feet toward the end of the table.

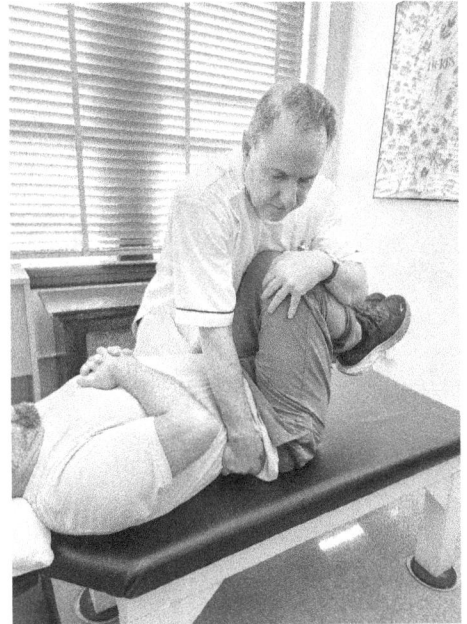

# SIJ #5    **Fulcrum Maneuver**

Site of restriction:  SI joint, posterior position or anterior position*

Patient position:  Supine

Technic:
1. Stand on contralateral side from the restricted sacroiliac.
2. Flex both legs and thighs.
3. Place both knees in your axilla.
4. Place other hand under the restricted PSIS.
5. Roll the patient over so that the weight of the pelvis and legs will come to bear on the fulcrum made by your hand.
6. Press downward on the patient's knees.

* If the ilium is anterior, place the contact hand under the sacrum instead.

# SIJ #6     **Supine Extension Release**

Site of restriction: SI joint, posterior position

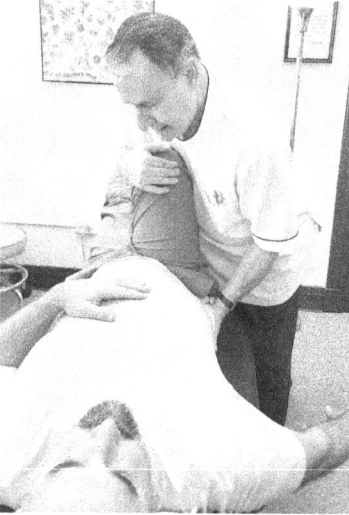

Patient position: Supine with thighs and legs flexed

Technic:
1. Stand on contralateral side from the restriction.
2. Place the close (contralateral) knee in your axilla.
3. Reach around his thigh to reach the ASIS.
4. Place other hand under the PSIS of the same side.
5. Have patient slowly extend the free leg and lower it to the table while you immobilize the pelvis with your hand holds.
6. Have patient repeat the movements several times until some increased motion in the joint is sensed.

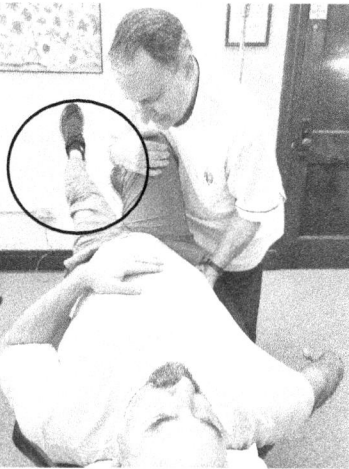

# SIJ #7     **Innominate Drop**

Site of restriction:  SI joint, posterior position or anterior position*

Patient position:  Supine with affected leg flexed

Technic:
1. Stand on ipsilateral side.
2. Position patient so that the entire innominate is off the edge of the table.
3. With the knee and hip fully flexed, clasp both hands over the knee.
4. Press down on the knee until any slack is eliminated.
5. Apply impulse downward through the axis of the femur, by dropping your weight suddenly.

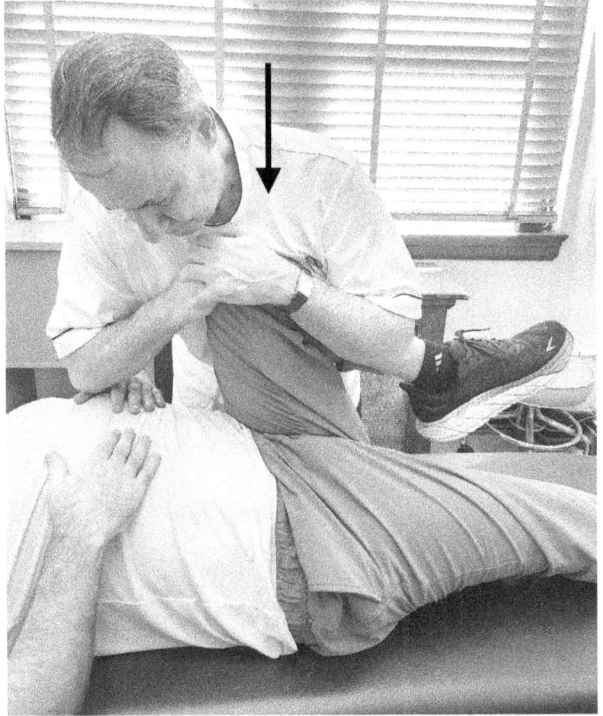

\* If the ilium is anterior, press the knee across so that it is over the contralateral ASIS before creating impulse.

# SIJ #8     **Prone P-A Maneuver**

Site of restriction:  SI joint, posterior position

Patient position:  Prone

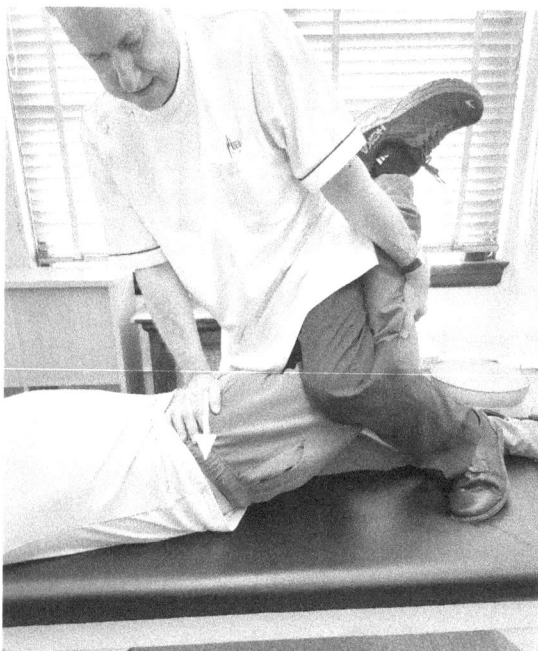

Technic:
1.Stand on contralateral side from the restriction.
2.Draw the patient's leg on the affected side over the other leg.
3.Hook your leg around patient's knee as in the illustration.
4.Place the hand on the side of the interlocking leg over the PSIS.
5.Place other hand over the contact hand and make several springing motions to move the ilium anteriorly.
6.Apply thrust to the PSIS, downward toward the table in a P-A plane.

**Abduction-Extension Maneuver**

Site of restriction: SI joint, posterior position or anterior position*

Patient position: Lateral recumbent on the unaffected side with the arm dropped off the side of the table.

Technic:
1. Stand behind patient. Position patient's legs in a flexed position.
2. Place your cephalic knee against the table to get your leverage and your hand on the same side against the PSIS.
3. Create a P-A pressure against the PSIS with your hand.
4. Grasp with your other hand the patient's knee on the affected side.
5. While maintaining pressure against the PSIS with your knee, use the hand to flex, abduct, and extend the leg. Ask patient to straighten the leg once it is in full flexion and abduction.

* If the ilium is anterior, perform the same except place your hand against the sacrum.

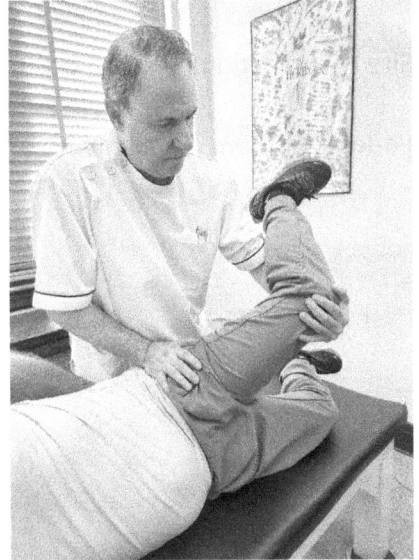

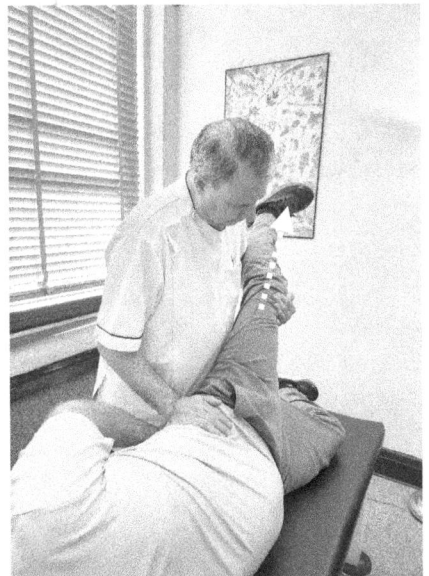

SIJ #10　　　**Longitudinal Leg Impulse**

Site of restriction:  SI joint, posterior position or anterior position*

Patient position:  Supine, with unaffected leg flexed

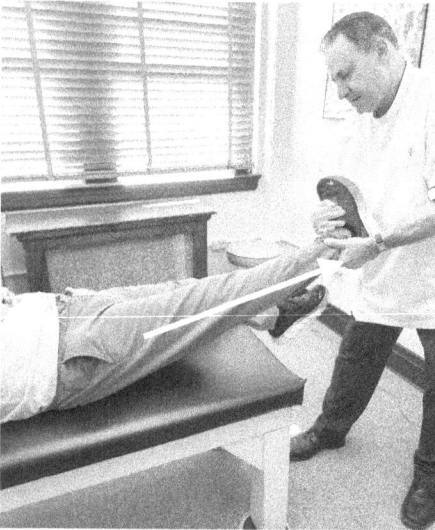

Technic:
1.Stand at the foot of the table.  Flex patient's leg on the unaffected side.
2.Grasp the ankle of the restricted side with both hands.
3.In extension, elevate the leg about six inches above the table.
4.Inwardly rotate the leg.
5.Tell patient to breathe in and out several times.
6.As patient exhales, pull the leg with a sudden jerk.

* If the ilium is anterior, perform the same but with the leg raised to 18 inches.

# SIJ #11    "Chicago" maneuver

Site of restriction:  SI joint, anterior position (in this illustration, the right side)

Patient position:  Supine with arms folded across chest

Technic:
1. Place patient's body in a bow shape with the convexity toward you (you should face a "smile", not a "frown".
2. Cross patient's legs (either one on top).
3. Face patient with your rear leg braced against the table.
4. Place your hand on the contralateral ASIS and the other hand grasps patient's posterior shoulder (superior and lateral to scapula).
5. Ask patient to inhale and exhale.
6. Toward the end of the exhalation, apply pressure to the ASIS in the direction of the sacrum.
7. Increasing the pressure on the ASIS, pull the shoulder so that the pelvis starts to rotate.
8. When the barrier has been reached, apply impulse downward through the ASIS.

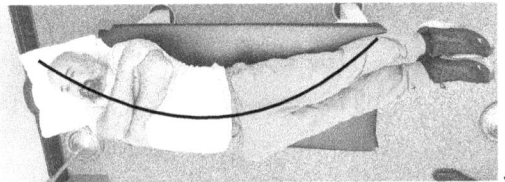

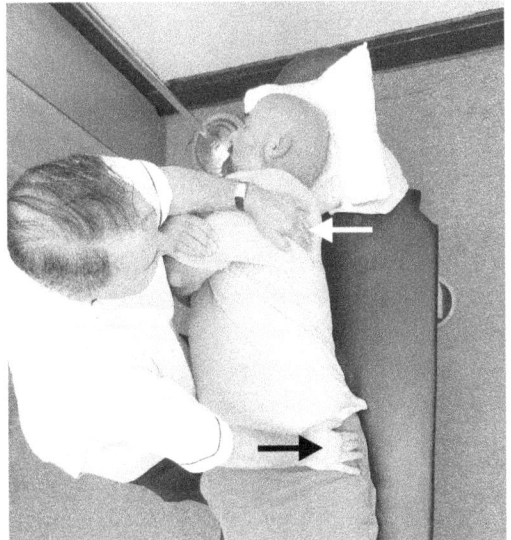

**Seated Sacral Torsion Maneuver**

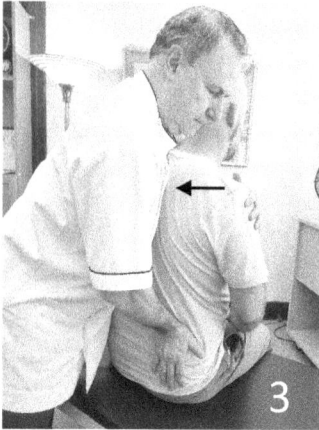

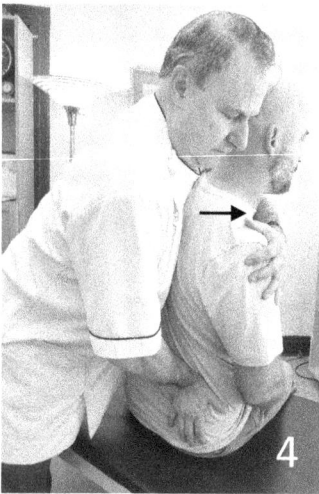

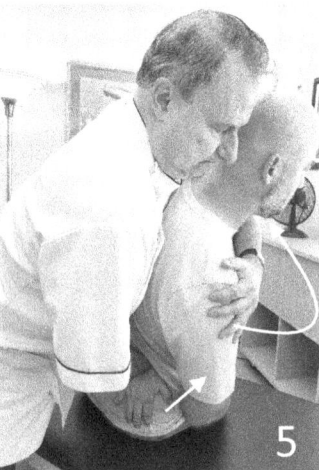

Site of restriction: SI joint, posterior position

Patient position: Seated, straddling the treatment table with the left hand grasping the right shoulder

Technic:

1. Stand on the left side with the left hand covering the patient's hand on the right shoulder.
2. Place the pisiform of the right hand against the right side of the sacrum base.
3. Induce a left side bending and right rotation of the torso, causing the sacrum to rotate left. Press firmly against the sacral base with the right hand.
4. Now reverse the rotation of the trunk to create right side bending and left rotation.
5. Perform a thrust P-A against the right side of the sacral base through the axis of your right forearm. At the same time create extension while side bending right and rotating left.

# SIJ #13     von Peters Maneuver

Originating with Dr. William von Peters of First National University of Naturopathy, it is included here by kind permission of Dr. von Peters

Site of restriction: SI joint. When the joint does not move either superiorly or inferiorly (likely an upslip), this maneuver is indicated. Low back pain that does not resolve from any other mobilization responds to this maneuver.

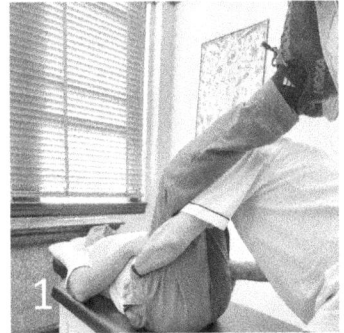

Patient position: Supine
Technic:

1. Stand at the foot of the table and position the patient's gluteals slightly off the edge of the table. Flex the legs and place them over your left shoulder.
2. Place left hand on the left ASIS, and the other hand on the contralateral ischium. The ischial tuberosity should fit against your pisiform.
3. Simultaneously create impulse downward toward the table on the ASIS, while making an impulse on the ischium, thrusting in a cephalic direction.
4. Make several thrusts, then switch patient's legs to your other shoulder, change hand positions and treat the other side, thrusting up on right ischium and thrusting the left ASIS down toward the table.

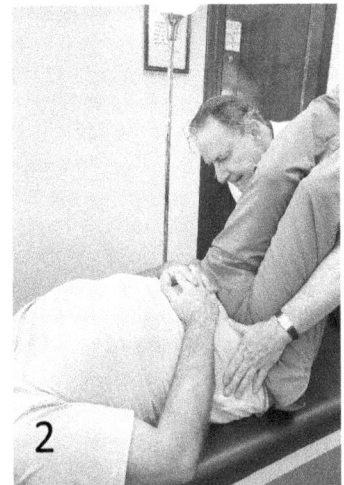

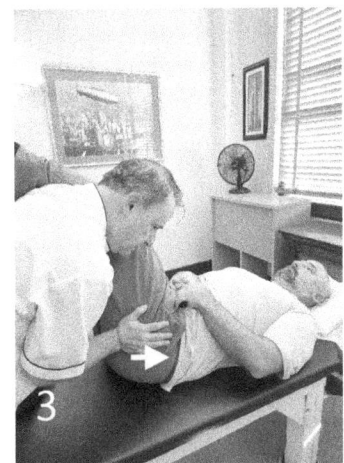

# SECTION SEVEN

## EXTREMITIES

### SHOULDER MOBILIZATIONS

---

## ASSESSMENT

**1. Check for reduced range of motion.**

  **a. Forward Flexion:** Have patient straighten arm
    and raise in front of him as high as possible.
    Make note of range of motion and any point
    at which pain occurs. Normal ROM is 180
    degrees.

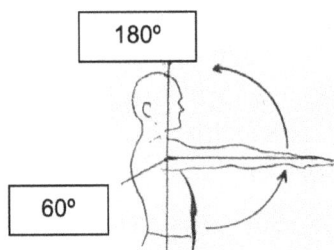

  **b. Backwards Extension:** Have patient reverse
    direction and extend arm as far as possible
    behind the back with the arm still straight.
    Normal ROM is 60 degrees.

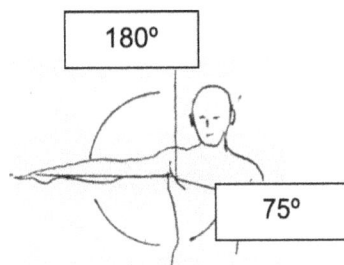

  **c. Abduction:** Ask patient to move the arm out to
    the side and as high as possible. Make note
    of any points along the range of motion
    where pain occurs, or the arm "gets stuck".
    Measure complete range. Normal ROM is
    180 degrees.

  **d. Adduction:** Have patient reach with straightened
    arm across the chest as far as possible and
    measure. Normal abduction is 75 degrees.
    Make note of any pain that occurs.

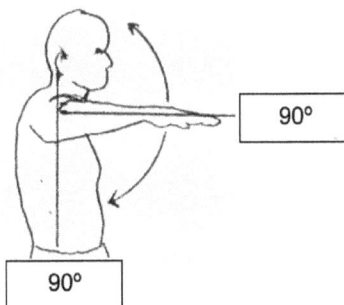

  **e. External Rotation:** Have patient abduct arm to
    90 degrees, bending the elbow, and then
    raise the hand as high as possible. Record
    the angle of maximum rotation. Normal
    rotation is 90 degrees.

  **f. Internal Rotation:** Have patient reverse direction,
    pointing the hand toward the floor. Record the angle of maximum rotation.
    Normal rotation is again 90 degrees.

## 2. Palpate the shoulder.

Check for shoulder tenderness on palpation.

**Tenderness over acromioclavicular (AC) joint** in absence of direct injury suggests arthritis of the joint. Have the patient shrug his shoulders as a test. Pain in the AC joint is increased by shrugging. Make note of a positive **shrug test**.

**Subacromial tenderness** suggests rotator cuff tendonitis or possibly calcific tendonitis.

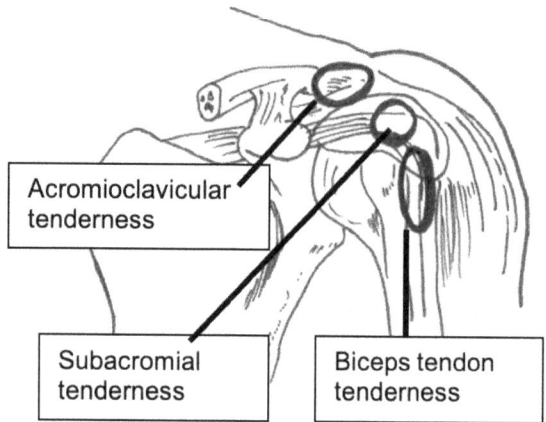

Acromioclavicular tenderness

Subacromial tenderness

Biceps tendon tenderness

**Swelling and redness** = inflammation of the capsule of the scapulohumeral joint (shoulder bursitis).

Acute bursitis usually resolves in 1-2 wks but many cases become chronic. Check for **Dawbarn's Sign**: If palpation of the acromial process is painful with arm relaxed, but not on abduction, it suggests subacromial bursitis.

If there is localized tenderness over the biceps, worse at night due to pressure from sleeping, it may be adhesive capsulitis. Tenderness over the long head of the biceps tendon suggests bicipital tendonitis. With the arm flexed 90 degrees, supination against resistance the pain.

If altered joint appearance or changed arm length, dislocation likely.

Note that Cardiac disease can cause shoulder pain.

## MOBILIZATION WITH IMPULSE

### SM-1

1. Knead the entire arm from shoulder to wrist, relaxing the subject.
2. Make firm squeezing movements with the arm supported so that the subject feels no need to hold the arm in position.
3. Next, gripping the wrist firmly, draw the arm superiorly and posteriorly (abducted at about 135º) at a pace that encourages the subject to be passive. When you encounter the resistive barrier, hold the traction on the arm. Support the subject with your knee in the position shown.
4. Next, pull the arm further while using the other hand to make a short thrust anteriorly, thus moving the joint past the restrictive barrier.

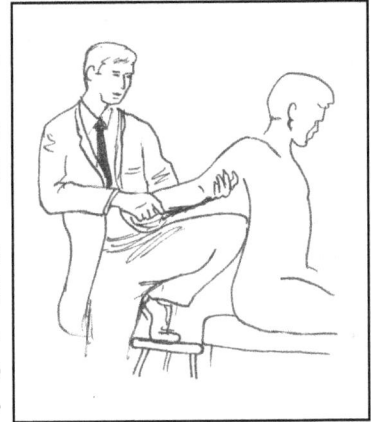

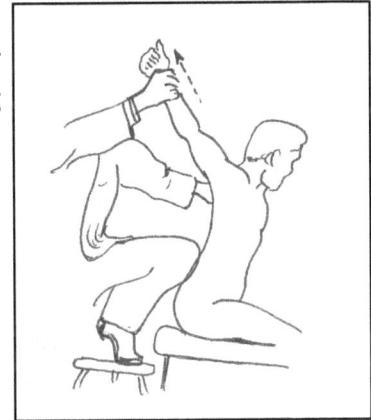

**SM-2**

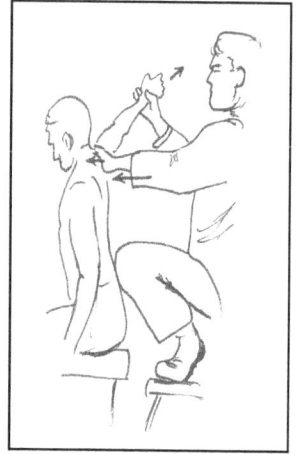

1.  In the same position as maneuver SM-1, but with the arm less abducted (about 150º), stretch the arm until a resistance is felt.
2.  Hold the stretch, place the other hand with the heel of the palm on the subject's trapezius and the fingers curled naturally over the SCM muscle, fingers pointing antero-inferiorly.
3.  Press firmly in an inferior direction without lessening the pull on the arm, then make a short thrust downward while pulling superiorly on the arm.

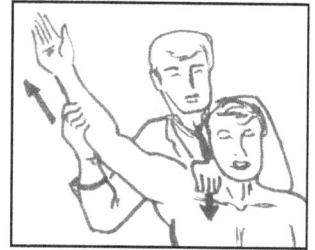

**SM-3**

1.  Grip the subject's arm just superior to the elbow, and draw it up and behind the head while it is flexed 90º. The upper arm should contact the ear.
2.  Pull the elbow toward the opposite shoulder, while maintaining a downward pressure on the opposite trapezius with your other hand.
3.  When the resistive barrier is met, hold that position for at least six seconds, then slowly lower the arm to the subject's side. Repeat if needed.

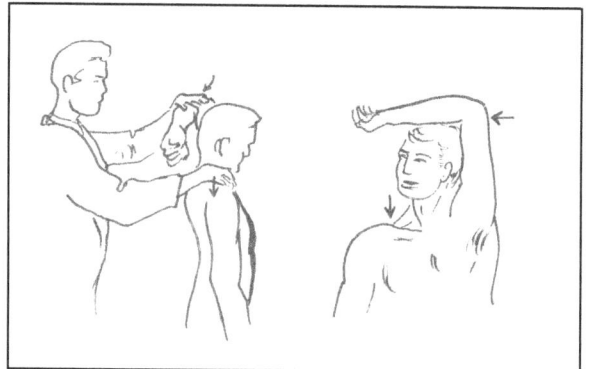

**SM-4**

1. Have the subject place the hand of the unaffected limb on the opposite shoulder.
2. From behind the subject, cup the elbow in your hand, pressing down on the trapezius with your other hand.
3. Now make a series of short thrusts in opposing directions with both hands, raising the shoulder by pulling the humerus superiorly while stabilizing the clavicle with the inferiorly-directed pressure.

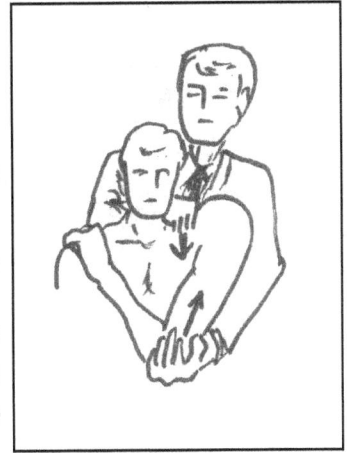

**SM-5      Rotator Cuff Maneuver**

This mobilization is for rotator cuff tendon impingement.

1. Have patient supine with affected arm flexed and the hand on the body, to create an angle that relaxes the tendon.  Use the thumb to make a firm contact under the tendon and press caudally.
2. While maintaining the thumb pressure, guide the arm through passive external rotation.  Keep the elbow at the same level and do not abduct the arm. The tendon will slip into position under your thumb.    Note: Discontinue procedure if strong pain is elicited.
3. Keeping a firm pressure with the thumb, extend the arm as seen in the illustration.

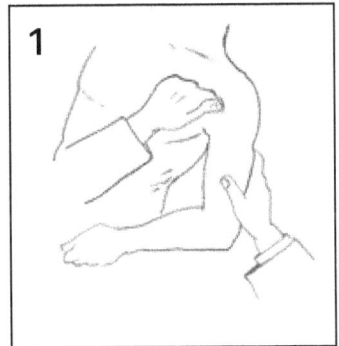

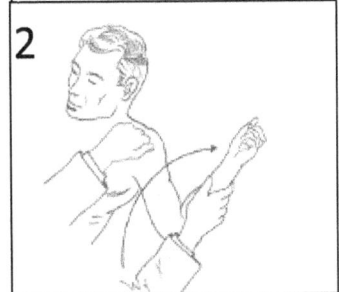

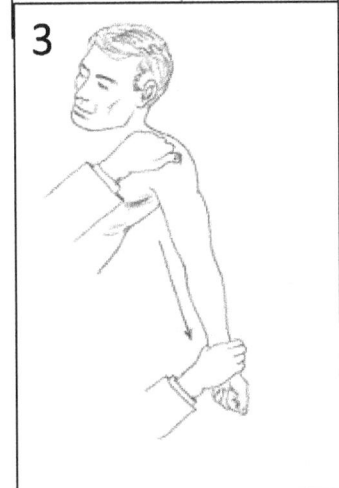

## ASSESSMENT

### 1. Range of Motion

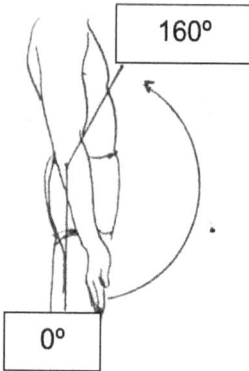

160°

0°

**a.  Extension and Flexion:**  Have the patient completely extend the arm at his side.  See if the arm goes to a neutral 0 degrees.  Next ask him to bend the elbow as far as possible.  Make note of the angle of flexion.    Normal ROM is 160 degrees.b. External and Internal Rotation:

**b.**  Have the patient place the ulnar surface of the hand on a table, and ask him to turn the palm up.  Supination or external rotation should measure 90 degrees.    Then ask him to turn the palm down and measure pronation or internal rotation.  This should also be 90 degrees.  Make note of the ROM in both planes.

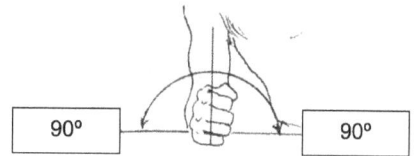

90°          90°

**ELBOW PAIN MAP**

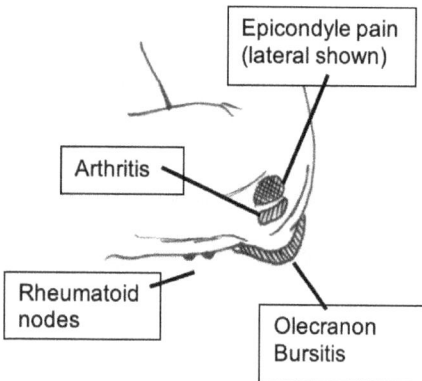

Epicondyle pain (lateral shown)

Arthritis

Rheumatoid nodes

Olecranon Bursitis

### 2. Palpation:

A tender, painful lateral epicondyle suggests *lateral epicondylitis* ("tennis elbow").    Pain is aggravated by dorsiflexion and supination of the wrist against resistance (Cozen's Test).

When occurring on the medial side (not illustrated), it is *medial epicondylitis* ("pitcher's elbow").  Pain is aggravated by flexion and pronation of the wrist against resistance.

Swelling and tenderness in the groove between the epicondyle and the olecranon process suggests **arthritis** of the elbow joint.

Swelling found superficial to the olecranon bursa, suggesting **olecranon bursitis**.

Subcutaneous non-tender nodules found in the elbow region occurring along the extensor surface are consistent with **rheumatoid nodes**. They are associated with rheumatoid arthritis.

## MOBILIZATION WITHOUT IMPULSE

**PNF**

Patient is supine. Stand at the side of the table and place patient's elbow into full extension, supine on the table. Ask patient to gently try to pronate the forearm against your resistance. Hold for four seconds, then have the patient relax. Make 3-4 repetitions.

## MOBILIZATION WITH IMPULSE

**EM-1**     **Abduction / Adduction Restriction Release**

Patient position: Seated
Technic:

1. Stand facing the patient and grasp his elbow. This will be the active hand.
2. The fingers of your hand should be on either side of the olecranon.
3. The other hand is used to stabilize the arm in extension / supination.
4. Assess the ROM of the radioulnar joint in adduction and abduction.
5. If a restriction is found in adduction, place the elbow into full extension and adduction, and make a corrective impulse to hyperadduct the joint.
6. If a restriction is found in abduction, place the elbow into full extension and abduction. Make a corrective impulse to hyperabduct the joint.

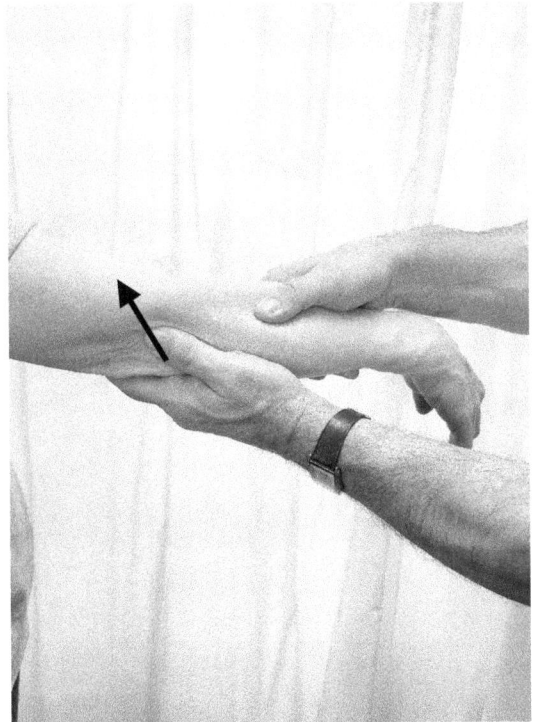

For radial head restriction

Patient position:  Seated
Technic:

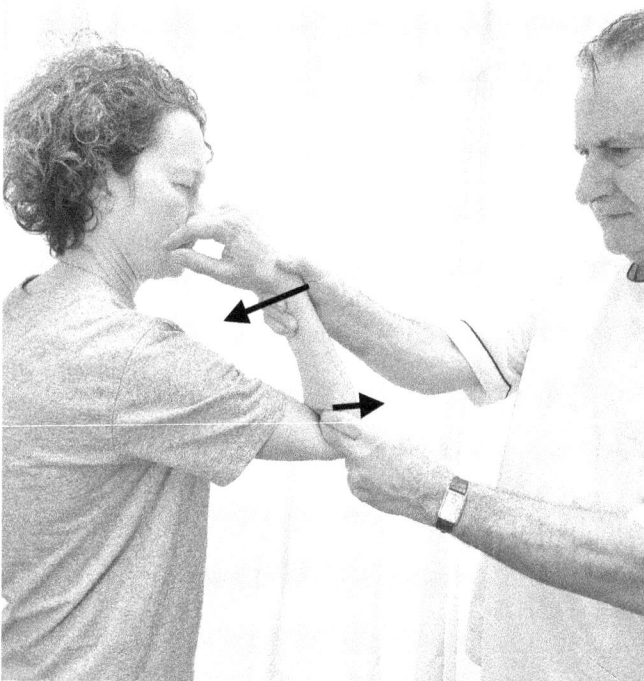

1.Stand facing the patient and flex the elbow while pronating the wrist.

2.Place the fingers of your other hand into the antecubital fossa over the radial head.

3.Make a rapid impulse to hyperflex the elbow and simultaneously thrust against the radial head with the fingers, in a dorsal direction.

It should be noted that a displaced radial head is one of the most common causes of elbow dysfunction.

## EM-3    Radioulnar Release

For radial head or ulnar styloid restriction

Patient position:  Supine

Technic:
1. Stand on the side of the table with patient's affected arm over the side.
2. Grasp the wrist of the affected arm with your legs, just above the knees.
3. Flex your knees slightly.
4. Grasp the elbow as seen with the fingers laced on the dorsal side and the thumbs placed firmly over the radial head or ulnar styloid as called for.
5. Quickly create a sudden upward impulse with the hands while straightening the knees.  The pull from the legs creates traction and the upward impulse releases the radioulnar joints by brief hyperextension.

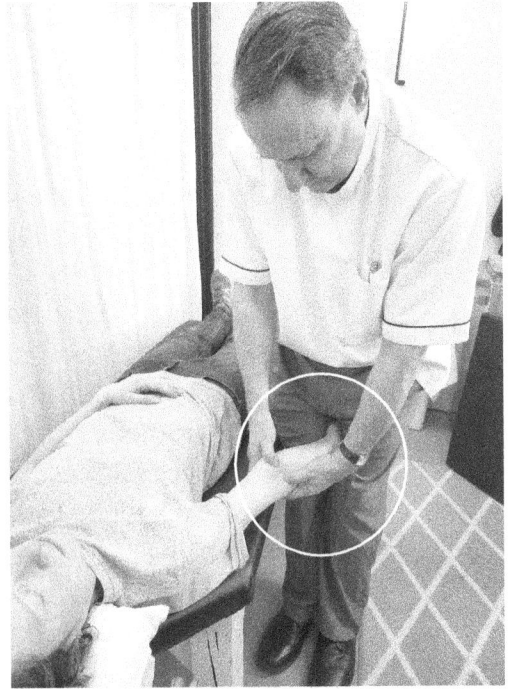

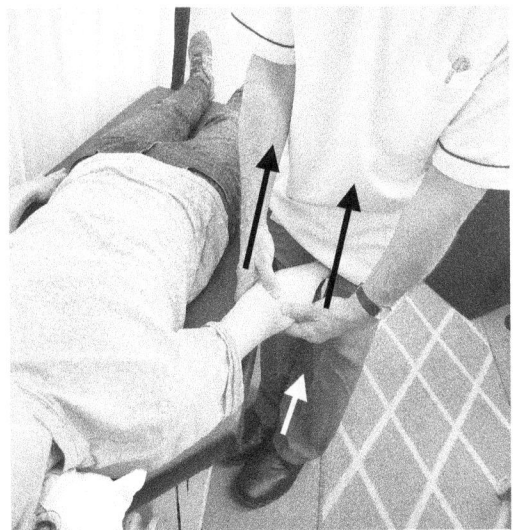

## ASSESSMENT

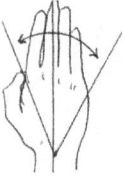

Normal wrist ROM ulnar flexion 45º
Normal wrist ROM radial flexion 45º

Normal wrist ROM flexion 90º
Normal wrist dorsiflexion 90º

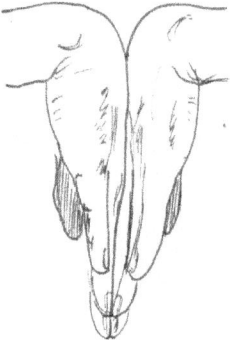

Phalen's Sign: Hold patient's wrists in flexion for 60 seconds. If numbness and paresthesia is felt over palmar surface, or fingers 1,2,3, and half of 4th finger, it is positive for Carpal Tunnel Syndrome.
Check for soft tissue restrictions in volar aspect of forearm.
Check for deviations in the cervical spine and paraspinal muscles.

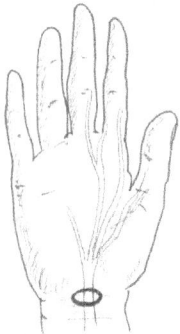

Tinel's Sign: Tap over median nerve on palmar surface of wrist. If tingling occurs there, it is (+) for CTS.
Check for fibrous nodules (myogeloses) in volar aspect of forearm.
Check for deviations in the cervical spine and paraspinal muscles.

## MOBILIZATION WITHOUT IMPULSE

**PNF**

Move patient's wrist into ulnar deviation until the barrier is felt. Then ask patient to push in a radial direction while you resist the movement. Hold for four seconds, then release the tension. Make 3-4 repetitions.

### HWM-1    Carpal Restriction Release

Patient position: Seated

Technic:

1. Stand facing the patient and grasp the affected hand with both hands, pronate it, and localize the dorsal radiocarpal joint with your thumbs.
2. Make a "crack the whip" motion, rapidly dorsiflexing the wrist while applying firm downward pressure to the distal ends of the radius and ulna.

Note: This same maneuver can be used for carpophalangeal restriction by simply placing the thumbs more distally on the row of carpal bones, and making the same impulse.

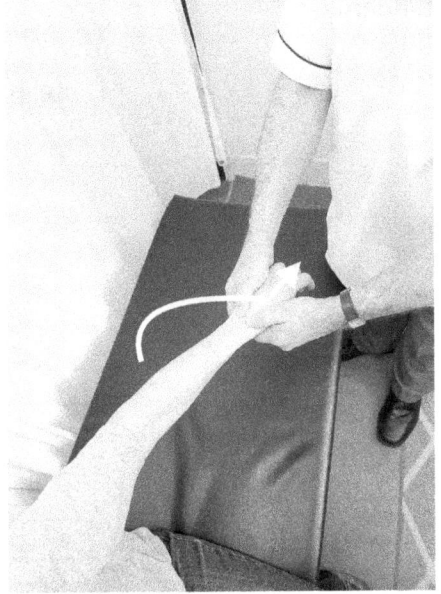

### HWM-2    Phalangeal Restriction Release

Patient position: Seated

Technic:

1. Stand facing the patient and hold the wrist to stabilize it.
2. Create a traction on the affected finger, and rapidly apply impulse to force the targeted joint into a gapping and brief hyperflexion, aided by movement of the finger below the phalax above the joint. In this illustration, the proximal joint is isolated, but the principle applies to any of the joints.

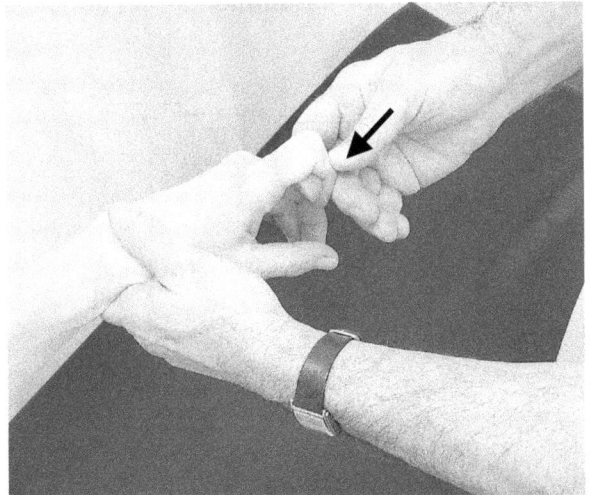

## ASSESSMENT

### Palpation

Palpate the fingers and note any abnormalities in size, angulation, discoloration, and tenderness.

MCP joints

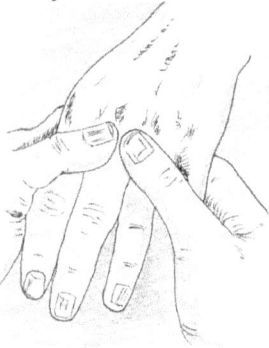

Distal phalanx

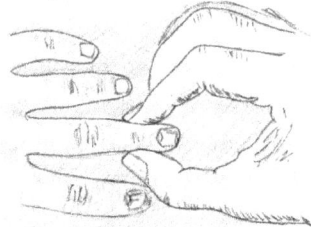

Check for texture changes and tenderness in the metacarpo-phalangeal (MCP) joints, the proximal interphalangeal (PIP) joints, and the distal interphalangeal (DIP) joints. Then check ROM of the thumb and fingers.

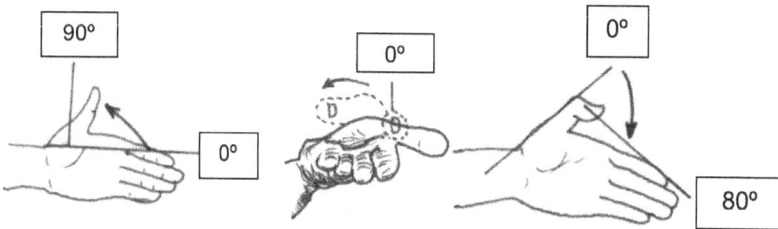

The thumb in (1) normal abduction, (2) adduction, (3) flexion of the IP joint

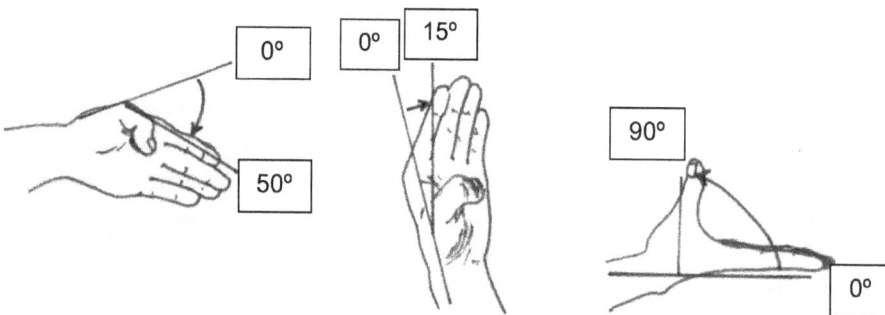

Extension (1) of the thumb MCP joint, (2) flexion of the CMC joint, and (3) circumduction of the fingers

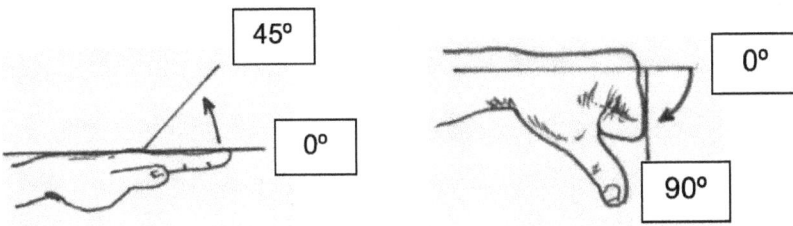

Extension (1) of the MCP joints, (2) flexion of the MCP joints

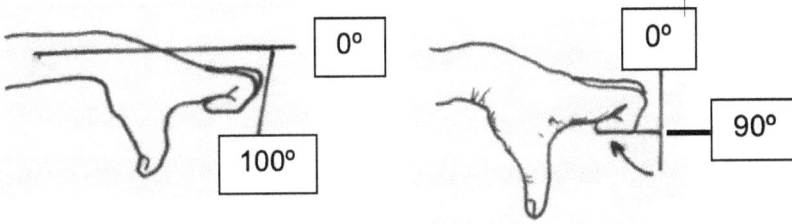

Flexion of the PIP joints (1) and flexion of the DIP joints (2)

## MOBILIZATION WITHOUT IMPULSE

Lock the restricted metacarpal between your thumb and index finger. With the other hand, use the thumb and index finger to maneuver the neighboring phalanx into anterior or posterior gliding motions, or rotation, if a barrier is felt to rotation. Use rhythmic oscillations.

## MOBILIZATION WITH IMPULSE

### FM-1    First Metacarpal Maneuver

Patient position:  Any
Technic:

1. Grasp patient's wrist with your cephalic hand and immobilize the carpal bones.
2. Hold the thumb with your other hand and pull it, creating traction on the CMC and MCP joints.
3. Now internally rotate the thumb.
4. With traction and rotation unchanging, use your thumbs to create a downward impulse over the MCP joint by quickly extending your arms.

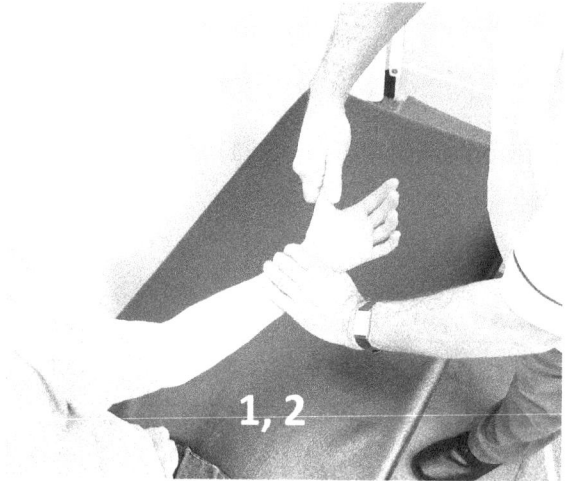

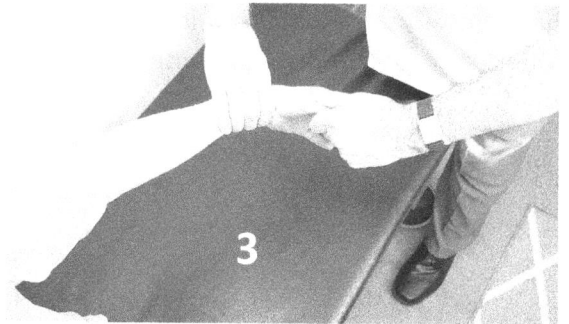

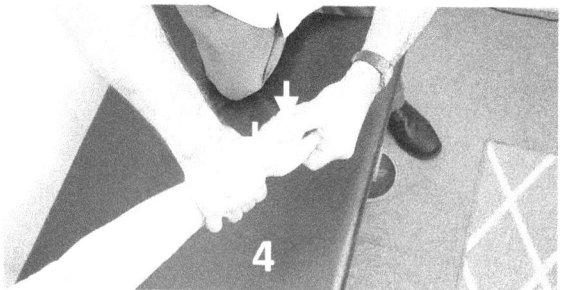

**Phalangeal Release**

Can be used to treat any finger, any joint.

Patient position: Any

Technic:

1. Stand facing patient.
2. Hold and stabilize patient's wrist with one hand.
3. With the other hand, grip proximal to the targeted joint and create traction.
4. Make a hyperflexion thrust through the restriction.

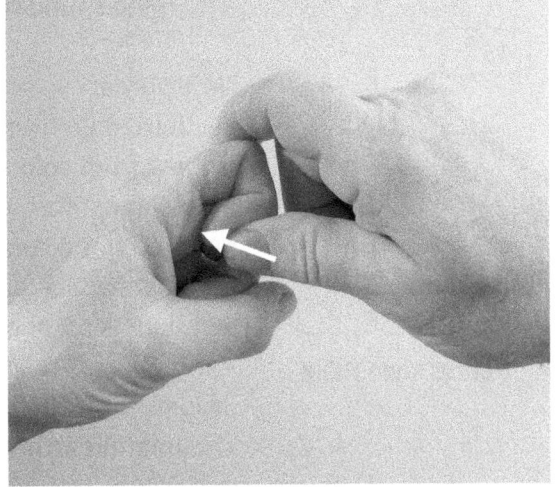

## ASSESSMENT

Before working on a knee, ask:  Was there trauma?  Was there a popping sound heard at the time of injury?

**No trauma:**
- Is there pain from damp or changes of weather,
- worse from cold, exercise or weight-bearing,
- transient stiffness worse on arising and from inactivity?
- Altered bone contours and crepitation on motion?
- Joint is swollen and tender but not warm?
- Patient is 55 or older?  It is likely osteoarthritis.

If joint is swollen and tender and also red and hot, it is likely rheumatoid arthritis.

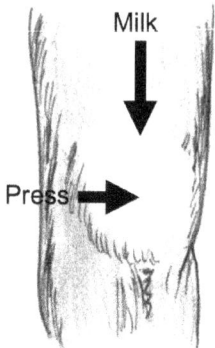

135°

10°

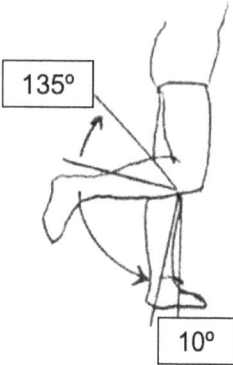

Normal knee ROM

**Traumatic injury:**
With patient supine and leg extended, squeeze and press distally the area superior to the patella, then with the other hand press directly on the patella with index finger.  If patella moves back and forth against resistance, there is effusion in joint.

History of sudden twisting injury with soft tissue swelling and possible discoloration, decreased ROM, and varying degrees of pain at different sites likely means sprain.

Milk

Press

# Ligaments

## 1. Drawer Test

To check for damage to the cruciate ligaments, perform the Drawer Test by placing the knee in 90º flexion, gripping the heads of the fibula and tibia posteriorly with the fingers, and pushing with the thumbs against the patella and femur while pulling the lower leg toward you.   Pain and/or excessive play in the knee indicate anterior cruciate injury.

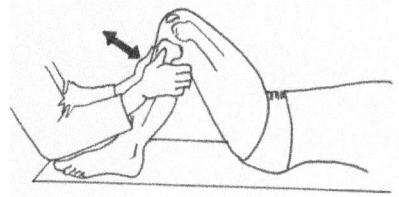

Reverse the directions to test the posterior cruciate.   Excess play and pain reveals an injury there.

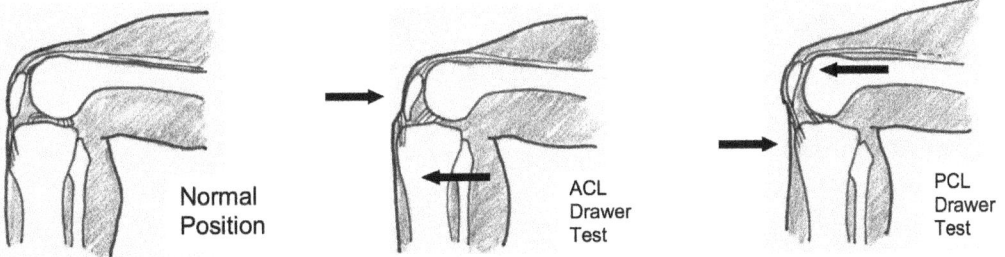

Normal Position

ACL Drawer Test

PCL Drawer Test

A positive Drawer Test indicates an unstable knee joint.  If Drawer Test is positive, and there is abnormal ROM, changed knee contour, fluid around joint, redness and swelling, there is likely ligamental tear.  Have patient lie supine with knees flexed at 90 degrees. Grasp the calf and pull toward you while pushing posteriorly on the patella.  Pain is a positive anterior cruciate ligament (ACL) drawer.  Then push on the tibial head while keeping the thigh from moving.  Pain is a positive posterior cruciate ligament (PCL) drawer.

## 2. Lateral / Medial Ligaments

To check for damage to the lateral ligaments, the valgus (lateral) manipulation is used.  With leg extended, displace the lower leg laterally while maintaining pressure in the opposite direction against the knee. Pain indicates a medial ligament tear.

To check for damage to the lateral ligaments, the varus (medial) manipulation is used.  Simply reverse the position of the hands to a mirror image of the illustration above, displacing the lower leg medially while maintaining pressure in the opposite direction against the knee. The leg should be in extension. Pain indicates a lateral ligament tear.

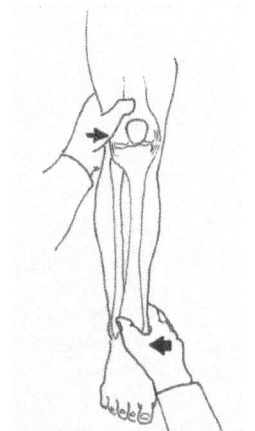

## Cartilage

Acute pain and localized tenderness and swelling, inability to completely extend knee, unequal knee contour, possible muscle atrophy of quadriceps muscle above knee, and a positive McMurray's Sign or a positive Apley sign, it is likely miniscal tear.

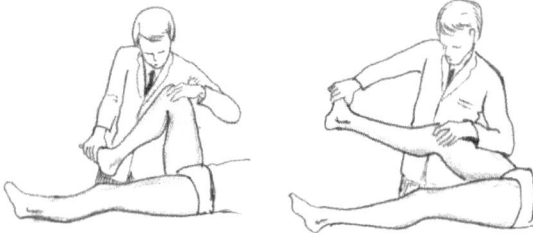

### 3. McMurray test:

To check for medial meniscus damage, flex the leg, anchor the thigh so the hip does not rotate, and then extend the patient's leg while externally rotating the foot. A palpable or audible click in the knee suggests medial meniscus damage. Performing the same maneuver, with internal rotation instead, tests the lateral meniscus.

### 4. Apley Compression Test:

When the patient complains of knee joint locking, apply the Apley Compression Test. Place patient prone and flex leg to 90 degrees. Press firmly on the heel, opposing the tibia to the femur. Then rotate the lower leg internally and externally in a grinding motion (also known as a "grind test"). Locking, clicks, or pain in the knee is a positive Apley sign and suggests a meniscal tear.

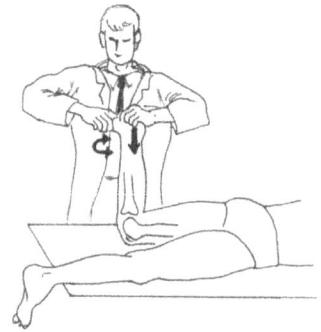

### 5. Fluid (effusion) Tests

To check for small to moderate fluid in knee joint, "milk" the knee in a superior direction to drain out any fluid. Then press behind lateral border of patella and watch for returning fluid.

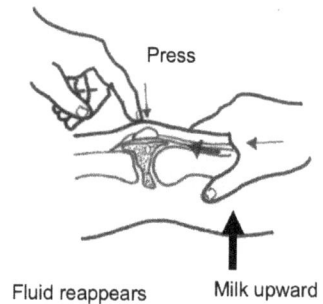

Fluid reappears    Milk upward

To check for a relatively large amount of effusion, compress the suprapatellar pouch (to drive fluid towards the patella) with one hand and with the other quickly push the patella back against the femur. If the patella moves backwards and forwards against resistance, or if a palpable click occurs, it indicates effusion in the joint.

# Differential Diagnosis for Knee Injuries

## CLINICAL SIGNS

| Site of Tear | ROM | Inspection | Palpation | Kinetic |
|---|---|---|---|---|
| Meniscus | Normal unless ↓ by large effusion or mechanical lock | Normal or slight to moderate effusion | Exquisitely tender along joint over affected meniscus | Positive click test on ballottement of patella |
| Medial ligament | Markedly ↓ by effusion and pain | Joint effusion, medial subcutaneous edema | Tenderness over medial ligament at joint line | Severe pain on valgus stress test. Knee stable in extension but unstable on weight-bearing, with joint flexed 15-20° |
| Anterior cruciate ligament | ↓ by effusion and pain | Tense effusion | Slight, diffuse tenderness | Unstable knee that moves forward on manipulation (positive drawer sign) |
| Medial and anterior cruciate ligaments | ↓ by effusion and pain | Joint effusion, subcutaneous edema | Tenderness over medial ligament and joint line | Pain and instability on valgus stress with knee fully extended; positive anterior drawer sign |
| Posterior cruciate ligament | Instability in knee posteriorly; effusion may make full extension impossible | Joint effusion, esp. in the popliteal fossa | Swelling and tenderness in the popliteal fossa | Pain and instability posteriorly with knee extended; positive posterior drawer sign |

# MOBILIZATION WITHOUT IMPULSE

A general mobilization for the knee is to have the patient seated on the table with the legs hanging free. Place an ankle weight on the affected leg and instruct the patient to make very small clockwise circles with his foot and to continue until told to stop. From time to time, the movements will become larger as he loses concentration, but caution the patient to reduce the circumference of the circles when that happens. After five minutes, have the patient make circles in a counter-clockwise direction in the same way for five more minutes.

# MOBILIZATION WITH IMPULSE

## KM-1    Medial Meniscus Maneuver

Patient position: Supine
Technic:

1. Stand at the side of the table. Grasp the ankle and place in your axilla (left side illustrated).

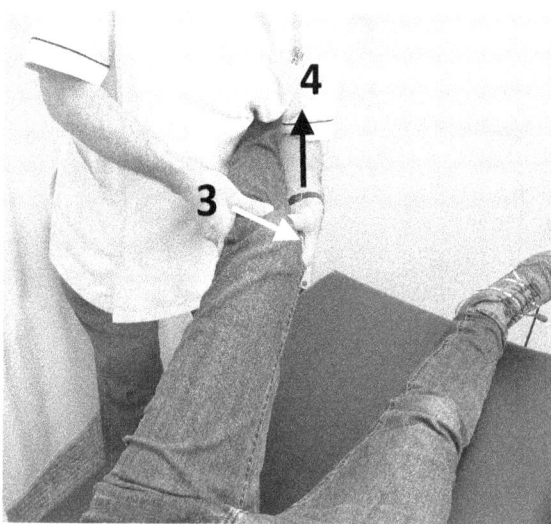

2. Flex the knee and hip, and place the left thumb on the anterior margin of the medial meniscus. Reinforce the grip with the right thumb placed on top of the left one. The fingers encircle the knee.

3. Press the knee medially across to the contralateral leg, causing a gapping of the medial side of the joint. Maintain this position.

4. Forcibly extend the knee while pressing firmly on the anterior margin of the meniscus. This will reduce the displacement of the medical meniscus.

## KM-2    Lateral Meniscus Maneuver

This is the same as the Medial Meniscus Maneuver, but with the direction reversed.
Patient position: Supine

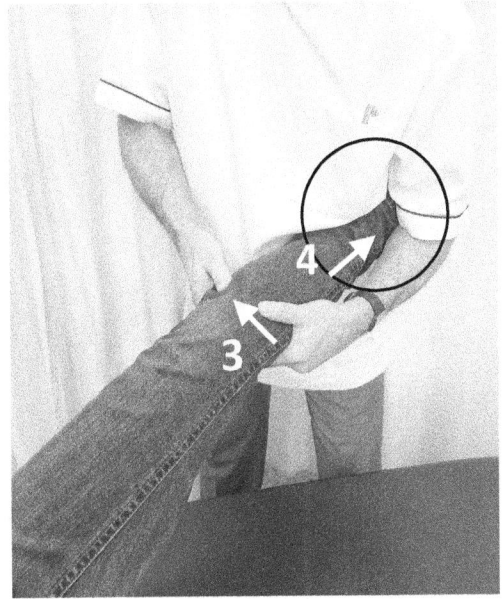

1. Stand at the side of the table.  Grasp the ankle and place in your axilla, as for the previous maneuver.
2. Flex the knee and hip, and place the right thumb on the anterior margin of the lateral meniscus.  Reinforce the grip with the left thumb placed on top of the right one.  The fingers encircle the knee.
3. Press the knee laterally away from the contralateral leg, causing a gapping of the lateral side of the joint.  Maintain this position.
4. Forcibly extend the knee while pressing firmly on the anterior margin of the meniscus.  This will reduce the displacement of the lateral meniscus.

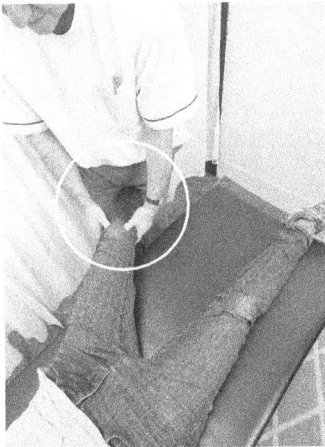

Variations:

Same procedures for the menisci but the ankle is gripped between the thighs instead of the axilla.

Or, you can be seated and drape the affected leg over your own, distracting the joint as needed (medical meniscus maneuver illustrated here).

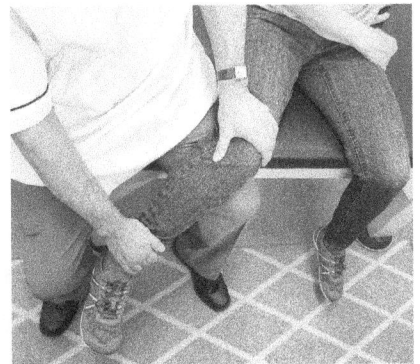

## KM-3    Posterior Tibia Maneuver

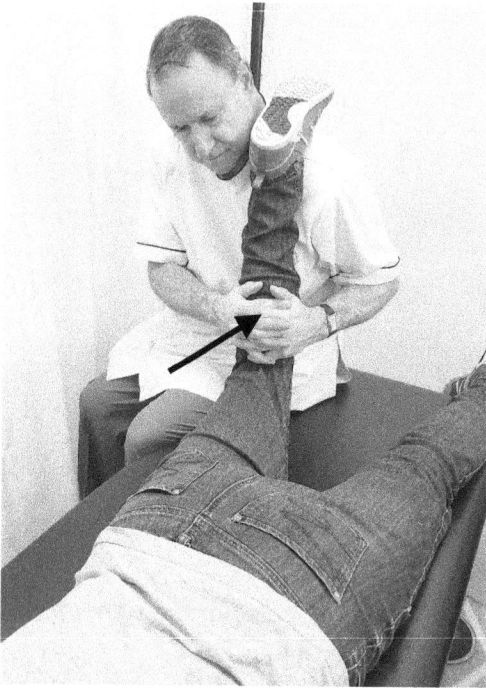

For posterior displacement of the tibia.

Patient position:    Prone with knee flexed ninety degrees.
Technic:
1.Stand at the foot of the table.
2.Clasp your fingers across the calf over the upper portion of the tibia.    Rest patient's ankle on your shoulder.
3.Suddenly pull the lower leg toward you in a longitudinal plane, moving the tibia into a more normal positioning.

## KM-4    Posterior Fibula Maneuver

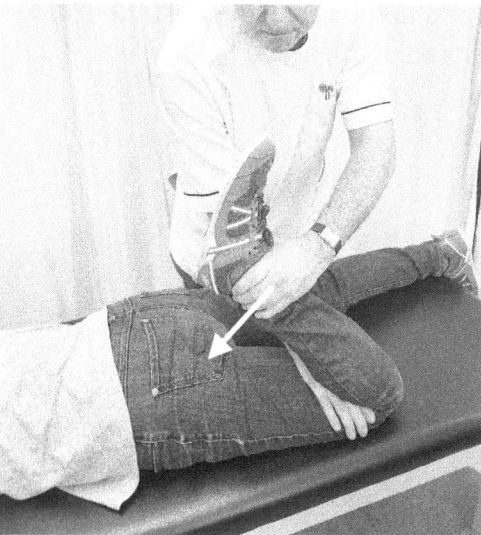

For a posterior displacement of the fibula.

Patient position:  Prone
Technic:
1.Stand at the side of the table opposite the affected knee.
2.Place one hand in the popliteal space so that is acts as a fulcrum when the knee is flexed.
3.Grasp the ankle so that the lower leg can be rotated by everting the foot.  This presses the fibula more firmly against the fulcrum.
4.Hyperflex the knee quickly against the fulcrum, causing an impulse that moves the fibula forward.

## ASSESSMENT

Check the ankle for range of motion in flexion and dorsiflexion. Normal ROM is 50 degrees flexion and 20 degrees dorsiflexion. Check to see if the patient can flex and dorsiflex against the resistance of your hand. Make note of any reduced range of motion or muscle strength.

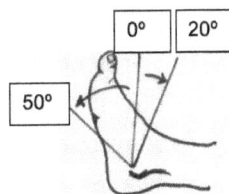

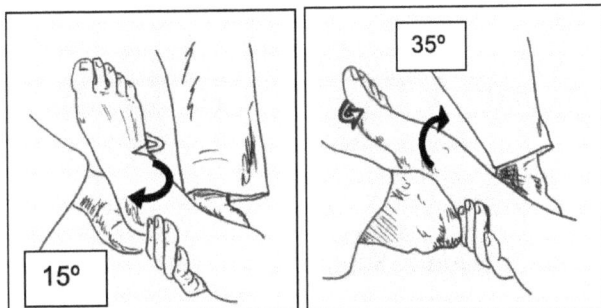

Anchoring the leg above the ankle, grip the heel and evert the ankle, measuring the degree of motion. There should be 15 degrees of eversion possible.

Anchoring the leg above the ankle, grip the heel and invert the ankle, measuring the degree of motion.

The sole should come up and the foot should be angled at 35 degrees.

Hold the foot in a 90º flexed position and ask Pt to curl toes, then to dorsiflex toes. Observe range of motion in both directions.

Record any restrictions to the joint that you find.

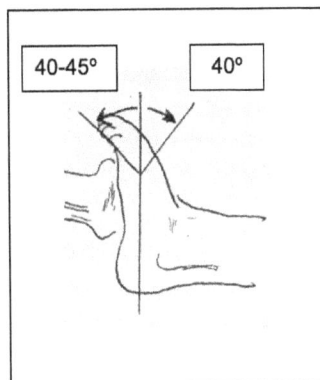

## MOBILIZATION WITHOUT IMPULSE

### Ankle Traction Maneuver

This is often corrective alone for any ankle joint dysfunction.

Patient position: Supine
Technic:
1. Stand at the side of the table.
2. Flex patient's lower leg onto the thigh, and flex the thigh onto the abdomen.

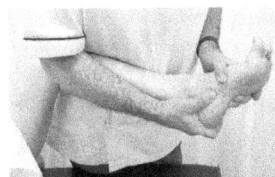

3. Drop the knee laterally enough to slip your closest elbow into the popliteal space.
4. The close hand grasps the back of the patient's heel, with the fingers under the lateral malleolus and the thumb inferior to the medial malleolus.
5. The opposite hand grasps the dorsum of the foot just distal to the ankle joint, thumb on the medial side over the arch.
6. Forcibly flex the thigh on the abdomen, while pressing the ankle toward the floor, keeping the wrist stiff.
7. With the other hand, now press downward to both maintain traction on the joint but preventing dorsiflexion.
8. Maintaining traction thusly, move the ankle through full range of motion in all planes.

## MOBILIZATION WITH IMPULSE

### AM-1    Long Axis Ankle Maneuver

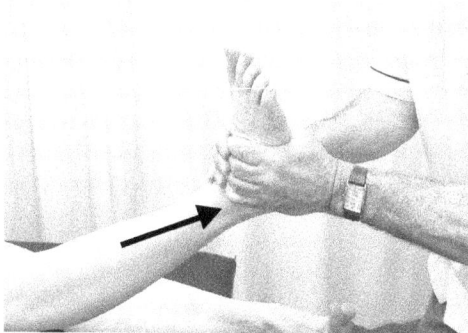

Patient position:  Supine
Technic:
1. Stand at the foot of the table.
2. Lace your fingers over the dorsum of the foot, distal to the ankle joint.  The thumbs are against the plantar surface of the foot.
3. Create mild traction on the leg.
4. Suddenly pull in a longitudinal direction.

### AM-2    Tibiocalcaneal Release

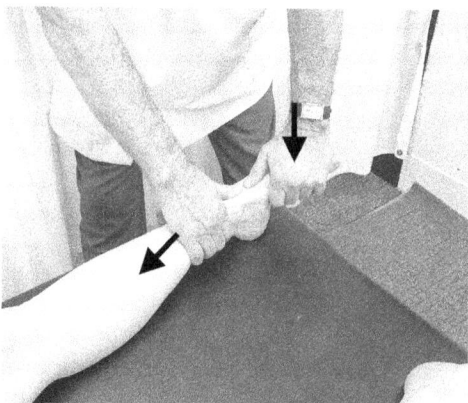

Patient position:  Supine
Technic:
1. Stand at the side of the table.
2. Cup the tibia and fibula with one hand and position the thenar eminence of the other hand on the dorsum of the foot.
3. Create traction by pulling the fibula and tibia in a cephalic direction, while the other hand keeps the foot immovable.
4. Make a rapid thrusting movement on the dorsum of the foot, toward the table while the traction is maintained.

## AM-3    Metatarsal Release

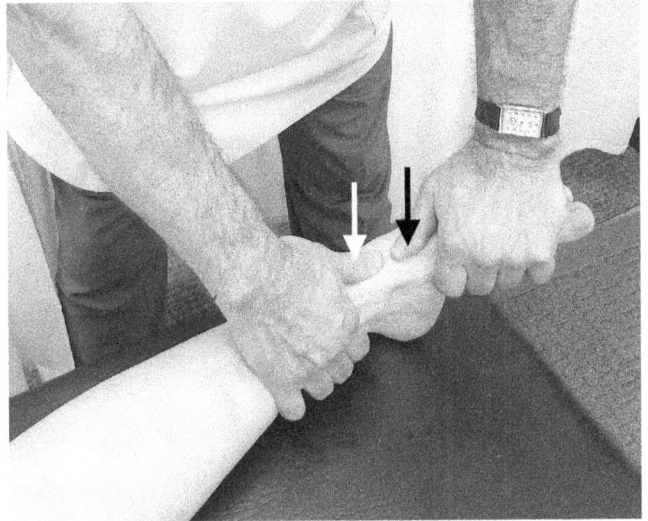

Patient position: Supine
Technic:
1. Stand at the side of the table.
2. Grasp the foot and place the thumbs facing each other at the site of whichever metatarsal joint is restricted (1st metatarsal illustrated). Each thumb presses on a different phalanx.
3. Thrust with the thumbs in a plantar direction, gapping the joint and releasing the articulation.

## AM-4    Transtarsal Release 1

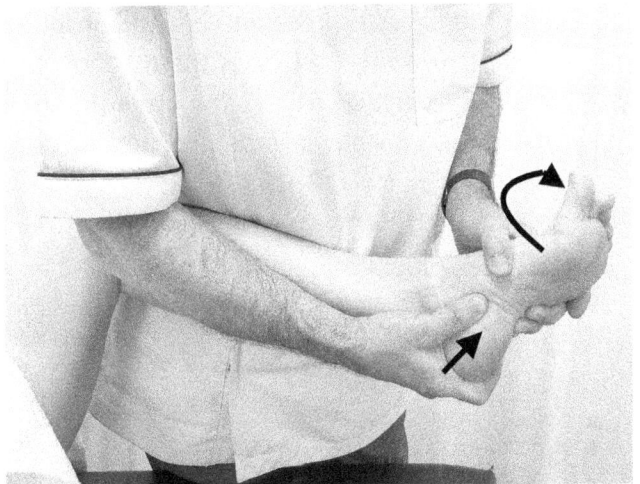

Patient position: Supine
Technic:
1. Stand at the side of the table.
2. Place the leg in flexion, abduction, and external rotation.
3. Place your cephalidad hand over the calcaneus, making contact with the thenar eminence.  Place the other hand over the 1st metatarsal and talus.
4. While twisting the foot into inversion, thrust down on the calcaneus with the cephalidad hand.

## AM-5    Transtarsal Release 2

Patient position:  Supine

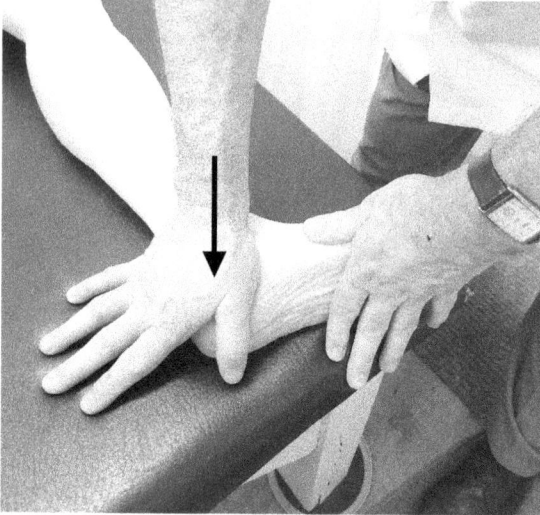

Technic:

1.Stand at side of table holding affected leg.

2.Flex patient's knee and place the lateral side of the foot against the table.

3.As in the illustration, create a rotational thrusting impulse through the two hands, holding the talus with your caudal and and making a thrust downward through the calcaneus with the other hand.


## AM-5    Cuboid-Navicular release

Patient position:  Prone

Technic:

1. Stand at the side of the table.
2. Flex the patient's knee and hip and drop the leg off the table.
3. Grasp the foot with both hands and place your thumbs in a V shape on the plantar surface over the cuboid or navicular, whichever is determined to be restricted.
4. Make a downward thrust with the thumbs while snapping the leg in a "crack the whip" motion.

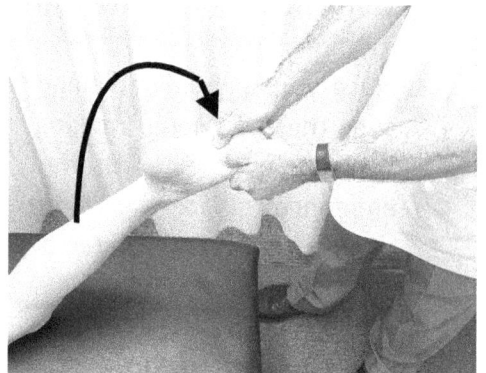

## MOBILIZATION WITHOUT IMPULSE

### PNF

Proprioceptive neuromuscular facilitation (PNF) of the temperomandibular joint relaxes the muscles of mastication and encourages better tracking of the joint.  Opening and closing, as well as side-to-side movement is challenged with resistance.

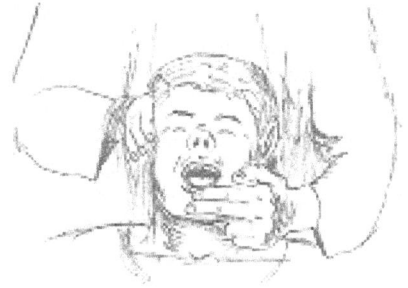

Patient position: Supine

Technic:
1. Stand at the head of the table.
2. Ask patient to open his mouth.   Place two fingers on patient's chin.   Ask him to try to close his mouth against your resistance for a period of 6 seconds. Perform 3 times.
3. Ask the patient to close his mouth.   Place two fingers on the chin again.  Now ask him to try to open the mouth while you resist the movement. Have him hold the tension for 6 seconds.  Repeat for a total of 3 times.

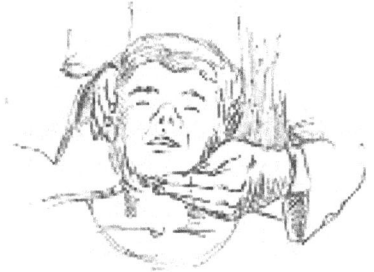

4. Now ask the patient to move his jaw away from the affected side.  Place two fingers on the side of the jaw, and ask him to move the jaw laterally against your fingers while you are again creating resistance.  Hold for 6 seconds, for 3 repetitions.

(Continued on next page)

## Counterstrain for the TMJ

Technic:

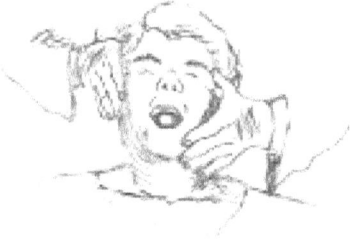

1.Palpate the TMJ and surrounding tissues. Find the most tender point (there will typically be one) with the patient's feedback. Keep the finger on this point with enough pressure to elicit mild pain.

2.Ask patient to relax his jaw and tell you when the tenderness at the point goes away. With the other hand, move his jaw toward the affected side slowly until the point is no longer tender.

3.Hold this position for 90 seconds. Then return the jaw to neutral position.

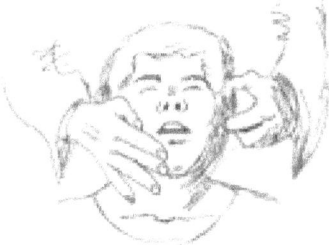

## Temporal muscle relaxation

Since the *temporalis* muscle is typically involved in TMJ cases, it is imperative to treat any reactive points in the area with digital pressure, acu-point therapy or Neuromuscular Therapy, etc. This muscle can be rapidly relaxed by use of mechanical vibration (Vibrotherapy).

## Suggested Reading List

- *Naturopathic Bloodless Surgery Technique with Treatment;* Paul Wendell, 1945
- *Greenman's Principles of Manual Medicine*; Lisa DeStephano, 4th Ed.,2011
- *An Osteopathic Approach to Diagnosis and Treatment*; DiGiovanna & Schiowits, 2nd Ed. 1997
- *Osteopathic and Chiropractic Techniques for Manual Therapists*; Michael, Gyer, and Davis, 1st Ed., 2017
- *The Teachings of Osteopathy As Given by Dr Andrew Taylor Still, MD, DO;* Frederick W. Collins, 1st Ed. 1924
- *Textbook of Orthopaedic Medicine, Vol. I: Diagnosis of Soft Tissue Lesions*; James Cyriax, 1975 (1947 under another title)
- *Textbook of Orthopaedic Medicine, Vol. II: Treatment by Manipulation and Deep Massage*; James Cyriax, 1965
- *Spinal Manipulation*; Bourdillon & Day, 4th Ed., 1987
- *Osteopathic Technics*; Samuel Rubinstein, Editor., 1st Ed. 1949
- *Osteopathic Mechanics*; Edythe Ashmore 1st Ed., 1915
- *Spears Painless System of Chiropractic*; Leo Spears, 1950
- *Chiropractic Technic Illustrated;* Michael Greco; 1st Ed., 1953
- *The Buxton Technological Course in Painless Chiropractic;* A.G.A. Buxton, 1st Ed.,1926
- *Technic and Practice of Chiropractic;* Joy Loban, 3rd Ed. 1920
- *Principles and Practice of Spinal Adjustment*; Arthur Forster 1915
- *Why Natural Therapies Work and How to Make Them Work Better*; C. P. Negri 2024

www.ingramcontent.com/pod-product-compliance
Lightning Source LLC
Chambersburg PA
CBHW080425270326

41929CB00018B/3168